# EAT 4 HEALTH

Katelyn
& Linda

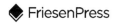 FriesenPress

Suite 300 - 990 Fort St
Victoria, BC, V8V 3K2
Canada

www.friesenpress.com

ISBN
978-1-5255-5967-9 (Hardcover)
978-1-5255-5968-6 (Paperback)
978-1-5255-5969-3 (eBook)

*1. COOKING, HEALTH & HEALING*

Distributed to the trade by The Ingram Book Company

# Eat 4 Health

# FOOD WAS NOT A FRIEND

---
### Katelyn's journey
---

Have you ever been told this about your health issues?

*It must be in your head—we can't find anything wrong*
*You must have picked up mould in your lungs where you were living*
*You must have frozen your lungs*
*You look too good to have any medical issues*
*You're depressed*
*You need counselling*
*You're allergic to your husband*

I'm here to tell you, it's not in your head. Foods we've been told for decades are healthy may be compromising our quality of life. And we continually make our health worse by the "healthy" food choices we make.

Food and I experienced a tumultuous relationship until I found the Plant Paradox program. Dr. Steven Gundry presented in *The Plant Paradox* that nightshade vegetables and grains, even gluten-free grains, have a defense mechanism for survival. They contain lectin, which incites chemical warfare in our body when ingested, causing inflammation.

Symptoms of inflammation in the body include:

- Brain fog
- Being on an emotional roller coaster, rethinking experiences and issues (like being in a video loop)
- Paranoia
- Zapped energy levels
- Constipation or loose stools
- Screaming stomach pains
- Stiff joints affecting mobility

I know I sure suffered for years. Let me tell you my story…

In my early 30s, I saw a natural nutritionist for many months and felt the best I had in years. My father was worried I was becoming anorexic because I'd lost so much weight. I felt and looked great, but at the time there weren't the grain replacement options that exist in the marketplace today. So it was very tough to maintain the diet regime the nutritionist gave me. I often said that life felt better without food.

I didn't understand the specific triggers; I felt like the canary in the coal mine. (My family heard me say that many times.)

My worst time came after working for five years in a very toxic hospital environment; my immune system became overloaded. Then we built a house I couldn't live in because of the toxicity of the new building materials.

I arrived at my deathbed, literally, and was informed I had three to six months to live. I was told to go home, do nothing and put my house in order. At the time I was diagnosed with an autoimmune disorder called Churg–Strauss syndrome. It caused major damage and scar tissue that affected my heart and lungs.

We had to make changes.

My husband Reg and I made a move to a rural BC community. We built a house using all non-toxic building materials and then started creating an organic vegetable/flower garden, herb garden, fruit orchard and a small vineyard.

All the explosions of vibrant colours, smells and tastes, all that diversity came into our kitchen, and life came to match the rhythm of the land with planning, planting, tending, reaping, harvesting and preserving. This journey provided the foundation for proper nutrition with nutrient-dense foods that became my journey toward better health.

In May 2017, a cardiologist told me I had an inoperable heart-value issue and that there was nothing they could do for it. If I had four regular heartbeats in a row, I thought I was having a good day. They wanted to try a few medications but needed the go-ahead from the respiratory physician. By November, they had tweaked enough doses that they were satisfied, and by December of that year, I was feeling considerably more hopeful.

Now, I tell you that little story to say that, if you need a pharmaceutical life jacket, for heaven's sakes put it on, but then get on with finding out what other changes you need to make in your lifestyle choices. In my opinion, the prescribing of antibiotics, acid reduction medication and cholesterol medications need some serious consideration because they disrupt your gut buddies and may hinder the absorption of proper nutrition.

Whether the Plant Paradox program found us or we found it, I'm not sure, but Dr. S. Gundry's thoughts challenged and inspired us. With the added body weight we both were carrying, Reg and I decided to make some significant changes in our food choices. We took the plunge in January 2018. The first week wasn't easy as we were both very much meat-and-potatoes folks. By the end of that year, we had lost a collective 100 pounds.

My sister, Linda, was living nearby that year and she joined us on our journey. Together we researched and modified recipe after recipe, and the result was this book.

The best news came when I saw my doctor after nine months of eating in this new way. He told me my blood work looked fantastic. I had been struggling with elevated white blood count, low protein, high cholesterol and high iron levels—indicators of poor nutrient absorption caused by inflammation in the intestines.

The results…

I have never slept better or felt higher energy levels. Now I live without digestive pain and bowel issues. My brain fog is gone, and my mental mood stays in more positive territory. I've discovered I have a total intolerance to all grains and dairy (casein A1).

Reg and I are very much a team in the kitchen. Many of our meals are last-minute preparation resulting in extremely fresh food. Reg brings joy and laughter to the kitchen. When I make flatbread chips, I score them into eight equal pie-shaped pieces. Reg adds neat geometric designs to his scoring. It lightens my spirit to laugh at the diversity we share.

Would I go back? Never!!!! The pluses far outweigh the foods we've put aside.

This cookbook may not be for everyone. But anyone who's experienced health issues that no one can seem to put a finger on will find help within these recipes.

These recipes allow the body to dial back inflammation. They let the immune system have a rest so it can get back to guarding the body. This is not a diet—it's a new way of eating for life.

---

**This book is written for those who want**
**grain-free, lectin-free, dairy-free, sugar-free and low animal protein**

---

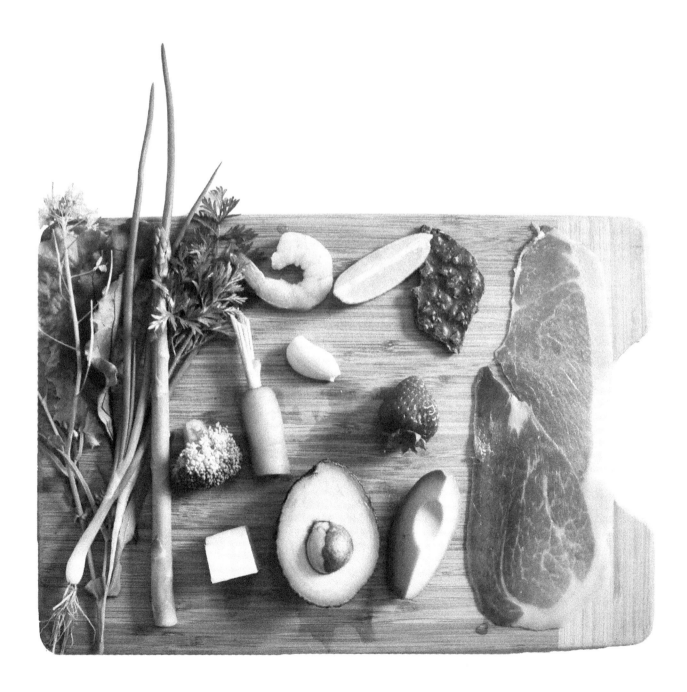

We recommend using only grass-fed, grass-finished meat and eggs

# THE PURPOSE OF FOOD IS TO FEED OUR GUT BUDDIES. WHEN WE MAKE A HOME FOR THEM, THEY HELP KEEP US AT OUR HEALTHIEST.

## So what foods feed our gut buddies?

Our gut buddies love fermented foods like sauerkraut, kimchi, pickled vegetables, cucumbers, carrots, beets, kohlrabi and whatever your mind imagines.

Foods from the brassica family help us fight bad gut bacteria. However, if you have a bowel disorder, you will need to eliminate these foods and reintroduce them slowly and well cooked.

Some foods our gut buddies love include:

- Mushrooms
- Dark Chocolate, at least 70%
- Green leafy vegetables like kale, Swiss chard, spinach and fresh sprouts especially broccoli and daikon radish
- Brassica family vegetables—broccoli, kale, cauliflower and Brussels sprouts
- Nuts and seeds like almonds, hazelnuts, macadamia nuts, pecans, walnuts, flax seed and hemp seed
- Fruits (in season only)—pears, apples and dark berries
- Onion and garlic

**Some special notes and tips about these recipes**

- In the following recipes, "GB" indicates exceptional gut-buddy food.
- All recipes use sea salt and organic ingredients.
- Yacon syrup can be used as an alternative sweetener in all recipes because it does not increase blood sugar levels.
- Garlic should be chopped or minced and allowed to rest for 10 to 15 minutes to let the medicinal properties to be at their most helpful.
- The Instant Pot is a programmable pressure cooker.
- Cross-referenced recipes are shown in italics.

# BEGIN CRITICAL THINKING

## Don't be swept along with the newest superfood

We need to learn to interrogate health information, to cut through the nonsense that's continually market-ed to us, starting with Canada's Food Guide. (Although, the recent changes have been a move in the right direction.) The industry has put far too much money into ideas, and then these ideas are sold to us as truth. We need to evaluate information and listen to our bodies.

We need to make better choices that directly impact our health. Cook at home to reduce the preservatives and chemicals in your diet and start shopping organic and buying grass-fed meats.

It's not what you're NOT eating (i.e., the newest superfood) that's keeping you from optimum health.

It's what you need to STOP eating—the processed foods, genetically modified organisms, grains, night-shade vegetables and dairy that are raising havoc with your immune system, creating inflammation and ill health.

**Take action**

1) Eat foods that feed your gut, particularly mushrooms and a variety of vegetables
2) Get moving! I recommend the Dr. Zach Bush four-minute workout (search for it on YouTube or Google)
3) Begin gardening to create your own nutrient-dense food
4) Get grounded in nature every day

# Table of Contents

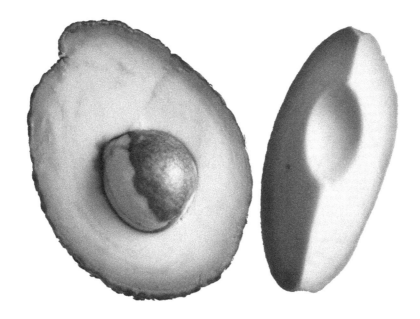

# Beans

## LECTINS ARE VERY HIGH IN BEANS

The good news - lectins can be reduced by proper preparation

By following the instructions in the bean recipe and you can enjoy your beans.

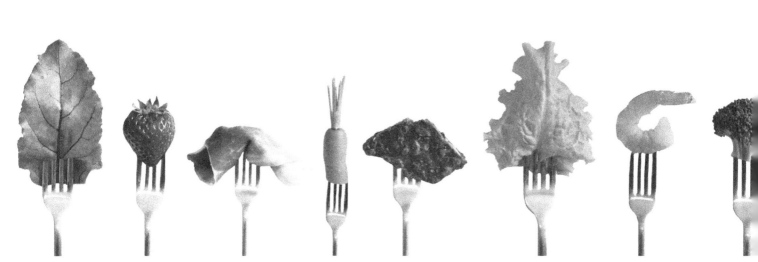

# KATELYN'S BAKED BEANS GB

|  | Prepare your beans by soaking in water for 24 hours: |
|---|---|
| 4 c | Mixed dried beans (adzuki, black beans, pinto, etc.) |
|  | Rinse at least three times to decrease lectin. |
|  | Once rinsed and drained, place the beans in an Instant Pot. |
| Add 6 c | Boiling water |
|  | Set the Instant Pot to 25 minutes. When it has completed its cycle, let the steam release naturally. Drain the beans and return them to the Instant Pot. |
| Add ½ c | Water |
|  | In a large frying pan, heat oil: |
| 1–2 T | Olive or avocado oil |
| Add 2 | Large onions, chopped |
| 6 | Garlic cloves, minced and rested |
|  | Sauté until tender and nicely browned. |
| Add 4 t | Dry mustard |
| 1 t | Regular mustard |
| 3 slices | Prosciutto ham, chopped |
| ⅓ c | Molasses |
| 2 t | Salt |
| 1 T | Balsamic vinegar |
| ⅔ c | Coconut sugar (to personal taste) |
| 4 c | *Katelyn's Tomato Sauce* |

Once remaining ingredients are added, bring to a boil and let it simmer
as the sauce thickens. Add the slurry to the beans in the Instant Pot and set the
pressure cooker for 20 minutes. Cook and let the steam release naturally.

Note: Pressure cooking destroys the majority of lectins except for grain lectins.

# Bread and Pastry

## COMING UP WITH BREAD RECIPES WAS CHALLENGING

The flours readily available today have resulted in some excellent recipe additions

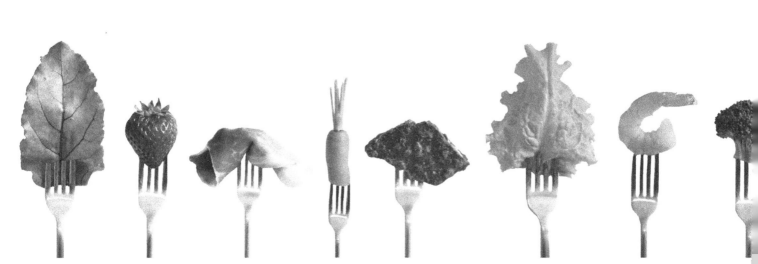

# BISCUITS

Preheat oven 400° | Makes 6 biscuits

In a large bowl, mix together:

| | |
|---|---|
| 1/2 c | Almond flour |
| 1/4 c | Arrowroot flour |
| ¼ c | Cassava flour (heaping) |
| 2 T | Flax meal |
| 1 t | Baking powder |
| ¼ t | Salt |

Add
2 T      Cold butter

Crumble the butter using a fork or knife, or with your fingers very gingerly.

In a small bowl, whisk until frothy:

3      Large egg whites (room temperature)

Fold egg whites into the biscuit mixture until blended and then refrigerate for 20 minutes.

Scoop 6 biscuits onto an oiled baking stone or pan.

Bake at 450° for 10 to 12 minutes until nicely browned.

Note:

A nice variation is to add 1/4 c parmesan cheese.

# BREAD & BUNS GB

Preheat oven 400° | Freezes well

In an electric mixer on low, stir all the dry ingredients together:

| | |
|---|---|
| 3 c | Almond flour |
| ½ c | Arrowroot flour |
| ¾ c | Cassava flour |
| 1 c | Psyllium husks |
| 1 c | Hemp seeds |
| ½ c | Ground flax (grind just before using) |
| 6 t | Baking powder (wheat-free, aluminum-free) |
| 1 t | Baking soda |
| 3 t | Salt |

In a bowl, whisk:

| | |
|---|---|
| 9 | Eggs (room temperature) |

Add
| | |
|---|---|
| ¼ c | Apple cider vinegar |

Stir together and add to the dry ingredients.
Slowly add into the mix:

| | |
|---|---|
| 3 c | Boiling water |

Continue to mix for at least 30 seconds until the psyllium has absorbed the water and the dough becomes sticky

The next steps depend on if you are making bread or buns.

**For bread**

Split the dough between two oiled bread pans. Let the dough rest for 5 minutes. Bake at 400° for 30 minutes and then at 350° for 35 minutes. Let the bread cool enough so the loaf releases naturally from the pan. Place the bread on a wire rack to cool completely.

Cut loaves in half and freeze, if desired.

**For buns**

Add
| | |
|---|---|
| ⅛ c | Apple cider |
| 1 c | Grated parmesan cheese |

Mix gently

Use an ice cream scoop or large spoon to scoop 18 large buns on 2 well-boiled baking stones greased with olive oil. Gently mould into a bun shape. Bake at 400° for 30 to 40 minutes, depending on the size of the buns.

Place buns on a wire rack to cool completely.

Note: Allow to cool completely before freezing.

# FLAX MEAL TORTILLAS GB

## Makes 4 golden tortillas

Place in a bowl:

1 c       Flax meal

Add

1 c       Very hot water

Stir constantly until the mixture becomes more gelatinous in texture.

Add

¼ c       Cassava flour

Mix well.

Cut dough into four sections. Place one piece of dough on a cassava-floured parchment paper and flatten into a circle with your fingers. Add a second parchment on top and roll out into a flat circle.

Heat oil in a skillet. Gently roll up the tortilla and then gingerly unroll it onto the skillet.

Cook until golden, and then flip and cook the other side.

Repeat the process to cook all 4 tortillas.

Note: These can be used as a delicious wrap or quesadillas.

# GRAIN-FREE PIE DOUGH

Preheat oven 350° | Makes a golden crust

In a food processor, combine:

| | |
|---|---|
| ¾ c | Almond flour |
| ¾ c | Cassava flour |
| 1 packet | Stevia |
| ¼ t | Baking powder |
| ¼ t | Salt |

Pulse to mix.

In a small mixing bowl, whisk together wet ingredients:

| | |
|---|---|
| 1 | Large egg |
| 2½ T | Softened butter or avocado oil |
| ½ t | Balsamic vinegar |

Add wet ingredients slowly to the dry ingredients in food processor as it is running slowly. Pulse for a minute and add water slowly until mixture is crumbly:

| | |
|---|---|
| 2 T | Cold water |

Turn dough onto a pastry pad and form into a ball.

**For chicken pot pie**

Cut ball into four equal parts. Flatten each piece with your hand, shaping it into a dough circle.

4 servings    *Chicken/Turkey Pot Pie Filling*

Divide chicken/turkey pot pie filling into four onion soup bowls. Gently place a piece of flattened dough on top of the filled bowls. Pierce dough with a fork.

Bake at 350° for 25 to 30 minutes, until the crusts are light brown.

# NO-GRAIN FLATBREAD

Preheat oven 350° | Makes 8 pieces

In a bowl, stir together:

| | |
|---|---|
| 2 T | Flax meal |
| 1 c | Almond flour |
| ½ c | Arrowroot flour |
| ½ c | Cassava flour |
| ½ t | Chili powder |
| ½ t | Paprika |
| ½ t | Salt |

In a separate bowl, whisk together:

| | |
|---|---|
| ¼ c | Avocado oil |
| 3 T | Water |
| 1 | Large egg |

Add to dry ingredients. Mix together well and form into a large ball.

Form into 1¼-inch balls (about 8 pieces) and place on a plate. Using a tortilla press, sandwich each ball between parchment paper and press into flat circles. Transfer each flatbread onto an oiled baking stone or other pan.

Score the dough with either a pizza cutter or pastry cutter.

Bake at 350° for 20 minutes until nice and brown.

For a variation substitute chili powder and paprika with:

| | |
|---|---|
| 1/2 t | rosemary |
| 1 t | oregano |
| 1 t | basil |
| 1 t | thyme |

# PIZZA DOUGH

Preheat oven 350° | 10 minutes

|        |                              |
|--------|------------------------------|
|        | In a bowl, combine:          |
| 1 c    | Almond flour                 |
| 1 c    | Cassava flour                |
| ½ t    | Baking soda                  |
| 1 T    | Oregano and basil            |
|        | In a small bowl, whisk:      |
| 2      | Eggs                         |
| Add    |                              |
| 3 T    | Olive oil                    |
| 1 t    | Minced garlic, rested        |
| 2 T    | Water                        |

Add to dry ingredients, and mix together. Allow the dough to rest about 5 minutes to firm up.

Form dough into a ball and slice it in half; create two pizzas or freeze one to be used later.

Oil a baking stone and roll out dough as thin as you can. Using parchment paper on top makes it easier to roll flat. Be patient as you roll the dough. Pinch the dough to create an edge all around. Bake dough for 10 minutes.

Mix together your pizza sauce ingredients:

**Pizza sauce**

|        |                              |
|--------|------------------------------|
| 1 c    | *Katelyn's Tomato Sauce*     |
| 1 T    | Pesto (or 1 t basil)         |
| 1 t    | Oregano                      |

Top pizza dough with the sauce and then your toppings:

**Toppings**

|        |                                              |
|--------|----------------------------------------------|
| 1 c    | Thinly sliced mushrooms                      |
| ½      | Red pepper, deseeded, peeled and thinly sliced |
| 1      | Red onion, very thinly sliced                |
| 1 c    | Spinach                                      |

Cover generously with shredded mozzarella and parmesan cheese.

Bake at 350° for 10 minutes, and then increase the heat to broil and brown the cheese.

# Dressings

## ACCORDING TO DR. S. GUNDRY

Cayenne, paprika and chili powder are the ground-up flesh of the pepper,
and chili flakes are seeds and skins (where most of the lectins reside)

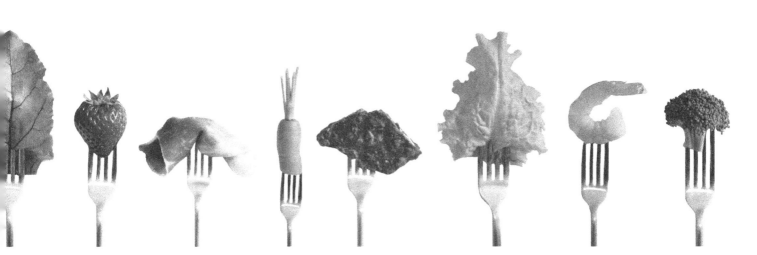

# BALSAMIC VINAIGRETTE DRESSING

## Fresh light dressing

In a blender, combine:

| | |
|---|---|
| 3 T | Balsamic vinegar |
| ½ T | Dijon mustard |
| 1 T | Maple syrup |
| 1 T | Minced shallots |

Blend well, slowly drizzling in:

| | |
|---|---|
| ½ c | Olive oil |

Note: Store in a jar in the fridge for up to a week.

# BASIC PEPPERCORN DRESSING

## Delightful peppery dressing

In a blender, combine:

| | |
|---|---|
| ½ c | Avocado mayonnaise |
| ½ c | Goat yogurt |
| 1 T | Pickled green peppercorns |
| 2 | Garlic cloves, minced and rested |
| ½ t | Worcestershire sauce |
| 2 drops | Hot sauce |
| 2 T | Grated Parmesan cheese |
| To taste | Salt and freshly ground black pepper |

Blend well, slowly drizzling in:

| | |
|---|---|
| ¼ c | Olive oil |

Gradually increase the speed to blend well.

Note: Store in a jar in the fridge for up to a week.

# COLESLAW DRESSING

Excellent cabbage slaw dressing

In a small jar, combine:

| | |
|---|---|
| ½ c | Avocado mayonnaise |
| 1 T | Coconut milk or goat yogurt |
| 1 T | Apple cider vinegar |
| ½ t | Coconut sugar (optional) |
| ¼ t | Paprika |
| ¼ t | Salt |
| ¼ t | Freshly ground black pepper |

Shake well to combine.

Note: Store in a jar in the fridge for up to a week.

# FETA CHEESE VINAIGRETTE

Greek dressing

In a blender, combine:

| | |
|---|---|
| ½ c | Feta cheese |
| 2 T | Sherry or red wine |
| 1 T | Oregano |

Blend well, slowly drizzling in:

| | |
|---|---|
| ½ c | Olive oil |

Serve over lettuce, peeled and sliced tomatoes, sliced red onion and olives.

Note: Store in a jar in the fridge for up to a week.

# LEMON CAPER DRESSING

***

Fresh tart taste

***

|        | In a blender, combine:                |
|--------|---------------------------------------|
| 2½ T   | Capers with juice                     |
| 2 T    | Minced shallots                       |
| 1 T    | Parsley                               |
|        | Juice of a lemon                      |
| 1 T    | Maple syrup or maple balsamic vinegar |
| ½ T    | Mustard                               |
| ¼ t    | Freshly ground black pepper           |

Blend well, slowly drizzling in:

| ½ c    | Olive oil                             |

Place in a jar.

Note: This dressing will keep for weeks.

# NELL'S JAZZY DRESSING

***

Sweet and sour

***

|        | In a jar, combine:   |
|--------|----------------------|
| 2 T    | Olive oil            |
| 2 T    | Coconut amino        |
| 2 T    | Balsamic vinegar     |
| 1 T    | Lime juice           |
| 1 T    | Coconut sugar        |

Shake well.

| Add    |                      |
| ½ t    | Celery seed          |
| 1 T    | Sesame seed          |
| ½ t    | Marjoram leaves      |
| ½ t    | Basil leaves         |

Shake well. Store in the fridge.

# RASPBERRY/BLACKBERRY DRESSING

## Delightfully fruity

In a blender, combine:

| | |
|---|---|
| 1 T | Dijon mustard |
| ¾ c | Raspberry or blackberry vinegar |
| 3 T | Maple syrup |

Blend well, slowly drizzling in:

| | |
|---|---|
| 1 c | Olive oil |

Shake well before using.

Note: Store in a jar in the fridge. It will keep for months.

# RASPBERRY/BLACKBERRY VINEGAR

## Requires patience but worth the wait

In a blender, combine:

| | |
|---|---|
| 4 c | Blackberries or raspberries (or a combination) |
| 3 c | Apple cider vinegar |

Pulse briefly.

Place berries and juice in a sterilized 2-quart jar and keep it on your counter for two weeks, stirring occasionally. Cover the jar with a fine cloth secured with a rubber band.

After 2 weeks, use a coffee filter or fine cheesecloth to strain the liquid from the berries. Lightly squeeze to get as much juice out as possible. (This does require patience but is well worth the wait.)

Pour liquid into a stainless steel pot.

Add
| | |
|---|---|
| 6 T | Coconut sugar |

Simmer mixture for 3 minutes uncovered. Pour vinegar into a storage jar.

Note: Stores a long time in the fridge - if sediment occurs on the bottom occurs just re-strain using using a coffee filter.

# RASPBERRY POPPYSEED DRESSING

## Light, refreshing summer dressing

In a blender, combine:

| | |
|---|---|
| 1 c | Raspberries |
| ¼ c | Coconut sugar or maple syrup |
| ⅓ c | Apple cider vinegar |
| 1 T | Red onion, grated |
| 1 T | Poppy seed |
| ½ t | Salt |
| 1 t | Dry mustard |

Blend well, slowly drizzling in:

| | |
|---|---|
| 1 c | Olive oil |

Shake well just before serving.

Note: Store in a jar in the fridge for a few weeks.

# SPICY SALAD DRESSING

## Spicy, warm taste

In a blender, combine:

| | |
|---|---|
| 1 c | Avocado mayonnaise |
| 2 T | *Sriracha Sauce* |
| 2 T | Red pepper, minced (deseeded and peeled) |
| 1 T | Parsley |
| 1 t | Dill weed |
| 1 t | Onion, grated |
| ¼ t | Salt |
| ¼ t | Freshly ground black pepper |

Blend well, slowly drizzling in:

| | |
|---|---|
| ¾ c | Olive oil |

Note: Store in a jar in the fridge for up to a week.

# YACON CIDER DRESSING

Tart and sugarless

In a blender, combine:

| | |
|---|---|
| ¼ c | Apple cider vinegar |
| 2 T | Yacon syrup |
| 2 t | Dijon mustard |
| 1 T | Red onion, grated |
| ¼ t | Freshly ground black pepper |

Blend well, slowly drizzling in:

| | |
|---|---|
| ¾ c | Olive oil |

Note: Makes one cup of dressing that will keep for weeks.

# Meats

## LEARN TO USE MEAT AS YOU WOULD A SPICE

### Add it for flavour

Research has shown there's a link between the groups of people around the world who live very long lives —they eat very little animal protein, if any at all.

Finding grass- or hay-finished beef and bison (instead of soy-, corn- or grain-fed) can help reduce the lectins in meats.

This may be crucial for those of us who are super sensitive to lectins in food.

Now a word about fats. Vegetable oils from seeds (for example, canola, corn or soy) are very high in omega-6s, and omega-6s are in most processed food. The link to chronic illnesses and inflammation is overwhelming.

Getting back to cooking with good fats, such as olive and avocado oils, and eating fish two to three times a week has been shown over and over again to be the right move.

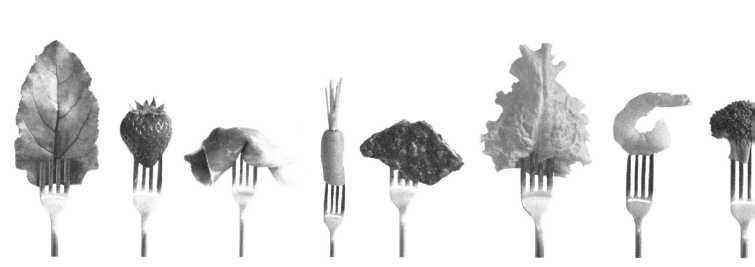

# BEEF & CABBAGE SCRAMBLE

## Quick, Easy and Delicious

|  | In a skillet, heat oil on medium-high: |
| 1 T | Olive oil |
| Add | |
| 1 lb | Ground beef (grass-finished) |
|  | Scramble hamburger until nicely browned. |
| Add | |
| 3–4 c | Cabbage, shredded |
| ½ | Red pepper, deseeded, peeled and chopped |
| 2 | Green onions, chopped |
| 1½ t | Garlic, minced and rested |
|  | Continue to cook until cabbage is nicely wilted. |
| Add | |
| 1½ T | Coconut amino (a soy replacement) |
| 1 T | Toasted sesame oil |
| 1 t | Ground ginger |
| Add | |
| To taste | Salt and freshly ground black pepper |

Serve with mashed turnips, carrots and roasted Brussels sprouts.

# BEEF STEW

Instant Pot

In a bag, combine:

| | |
|---|---|
| 2 T | Cassava flour |
| ½ t | Salt |
| ½ t | Freshly ground black pepper |
| ½ lb | Stewing beef, cut into small pieces |

Shake to coat well.

Turn an Instant Pot to "sauté" and cook:

| | |
|---|---|
| 3 T | Olive oil |
| 1 | Medium onion, chopped |
| 1 | Garlic clove, chopped and rested |

Add the coated beef and the following ingredients:

| | |
|---|---|
| 1 T | Coconut amino |
| 1 T | Worcestershire sauce |
| ½ t | Thyme |
| 1 | Bay leaf |
| 2 | Carrots, peeled and chopped |
| ½ | Turnip, peeled and chopped |
| 2 | Parsnips, peeled and sliced |
| 1 | Sweet potato, peeled and diced |
| 3 c | Water |

Sauté and brown well. Turn the Instant Pot to "meat" and add 10 minutes. Let it pressure up and cook; allow steam to release naturally.

Note: Daikon radish is a nice alternative.

# BEEF STROGANOFF GB

## Serve with Spinach Cauliflower Risotto*

| | |
|---|---|
| 2 | Beef or bison chuck steaks |
| | Cut the meat from the bone and remove gristle. Cut meat into small pieces. |
| | Sprinkle all sides of the meat with cassava flour. |
| | Combine in a pressure cooker: |
| 2 T | Olive oil |
| 1 | Medium onion, chopped |
| | Using the Instant Pot saute setting, sauté onions until nicely browned. Add coated meat and brown well. |
| Add | |
| ½ t | Salt |
| ½ t | Freshly ground black pepper |
| 1 c | Mushrooms, chopped |
| ½ c | Beef or chicken broth |
| | Close the lid and pressure cook on medium-high heat for 12 to 15 minutes to brown the mixture. Release the pressure. |
| Add | |
| 1 T | Cassava flour |
| ½ c | Goat yogurt |
| | Allow to simmer to thicken for a few minutes, stirring frequently. |
| Add | |
| 1 T | Parsley |

* Recipe in *The Plant Paradox Quick and Easy* by Dr. Steven Gundry

# BISON CHILI

## Serve with buns | 1 hour

In a saucepan, heat oil:

| | |
|---|---|
| 1 T | Olive oil |

Add
| | |
|---|---|
| 1 lb | Bison hamburger (or grass-finished beef) |
| 1 c | Onions, chopped |
| 3 | Garlic cloves, minced and rested |
| ½ | Red pepper, deseeded, peeled and chopped |

Cook until nicely browned, stirring frequently.

Add
| | |
|---|---|
| ½ jar | *Katelyn's Tomato Sauce* |
| 1–2 T | Chili powder (to taste) |
| 1 t | Salt |

Bring to a boil. Reduce heat and let simmer one hour.

Add
| | |
|---|---|
| 2 c | *Katelyn's Baked Beans* |

Cook until warm. Top with shredded cheddar cheese, minced onions and goat yogurt, and serve.

Add a large garden salad, avocado and bread buns to your meal.

# DEER STEAK FRIED

## Serve with mayo-less coleslaw and yam fries

Important: Remove from the meat any thin skin membrane, gristle, fat or bone. The wild taste from these will taint the meat.

| | |
|---|---|
| 2 | Deer steaks (meat removed from bone and sliced into chunks) |
| | In a bowl, whisk together: |
| ¼ c | Olive oil |
| ¼ c | Goat yogurt |
| Add | |
| ¼ c | Coconut aminos |
| ½ c | Onion, finely chopped |
| 2 | Garlic cloves, minced and rested |
| 1 T | Parsley |
| ½ t | Celery seed |
| ¼ t | Paprika |
| 1 t | Salt |
| ¼ t | Freshly ground black pepper |
| | Put on a plate: |
| 2 T | Cassava flour |
| | Roll one piece of meat at a time in the bowl of liquid, and then dredge in cassava flour. |
| | In a frying pan, heat oil on medium-high: |
| 1 T | Coconut oil |
| 2 T | Olive oil |
| | Drop coated meat into the pan and cook, browning well. |

# MAUI SHORT RIBS

Instant Pot | 25 minutes

Place in an Instant Pot:

| | |
|---|---|
| 3 lb | Beef or bison ribs |
| To taste | Freshly ground black pepper |

Turn the Instant Pot to "sauté" and cook the ribs until browned well on all sides.

In a small bowl, combine:

| | |
|---|---|
| ½ c | Coconut amino |
| ⅛ c | Coconut sugar |
| 3 | Garlic cloves, minced and rested |
| 2 T | Fresh ginger, minced |
| 1 T | Toasted sesame oil |
| ½ c | Crushed pineapple |
| ¼ c | Chicken broth |

Whisk together and pour over the ribs.

Turn the Instant Pot to "meat" and add time to equal 25 minutes. Let the steam release naturally.

Serve with Miracle Noodle rice, garden salad, and carrots or *Celeriac Roasted with Yogurt Dressing*.

# MEATLOAF ALL-IN-ONE

## Pressure cooker | 10 minutes

|  | In a bowl, combine: |
|---|---|
| 2 T | Goat yogurt |
| 1 | Egg |

In an S-blade food processor, mince:

| ½ c | Onion, chopped |
|---|---|
| 2 | Garlic cloves, minced |
| 4 T | Carrots, chopped |
| 2 T | Celery, chopped |
| 1 T | Parsley |
| 2 T | Flax meal |

Add all of the above to:

| 1 lb | Ground bison or beef |
|---|---|
| 1 | Bread bun or thick slice of bread, crumbled |
| 3 T | *Katelyn's Tomato Sauce* |

| Add |  |
|---|---|
| 1 t | Mustard |
| 1 t | Basil |
| 1 t | Oregano |
| To taste | Salt and freshly ground black pepper |

Mix well.

Place meatloaf in a baking dish that fits inside the pressure cooker on a rack with ¾ cup water in the bottom of the pressure cooker.

Spread on top of the meatloaf:

| ¼ c | *Katelyn's Tomato Sauce* |
|---|---|

Around the sides, add quartered sweet potato and four whole carrots.

Lightly cover the meatloaf with some tin foil. Put pressure cooker on "meat" and then add 10 minutes. Let the steam release naturally.

# SPAGHETTI & MEATBALLS

## Miracle Noodle dish

Prepare Miracle Noodle spaghetti as directed and set aside.

In a bowl, combine:

| | |
|---|---|
| 1 lb | Ground bison, beef or turkey |
| 1 | Bread bun or thick slice of bread, crumbled in food processor |
| 1 | Egg |
| 2 T | *Katelyn's Tomato Sauce* |
| 1 t | Mustard |
| ½ | Small red onion, finely chopped |
| ½ t | Oregano |
| 1 T | Worcestershire sauce |
| 2 | Garlic cloves, minced and rested |
| ¼ t | Salt |
| ¼ t | Freshly ground black pepper |

Form into balls.

In a frying pan, heat oil:

| | |
|---|---|
| 2 T | Olive oil |

Drop balls into frying pan and cook to brown well on all sides.
Set meatballs aside.

Add to the pan:

| | |
|---|---|
| 2 T | Olive oil |
| ½ | Small red onion, finely chopped |
| 1 | Garlic clove, minced and rested |

Cook until onions are soft.

Add

| | |
|---|---|
| 1½ c | *Katelyn's Tomato Sauce* |
| 1 t | Coconut sugar |
| 2 T | Parsley |
| 1 t | Oregano |
| ½ t | Salt |
| ¼ t | Freshly ground black pepper |
| 1 | Bay leaf |

Place meatballs in the sauce and simmer. Prepare the Miracle Noodle spaghetti as directed (pg.45), add the meatballs and sauce to the pot and blend well.

Serve with a salad and *Refrigerator Beet Pickles*.

# SPICY CHEESE GROUND BISON GB

## Preheat oven 375° | Great with pickled beets

|  | In a large skillet, heat oil on medium-high: |
|---|---|
| 1 T | Olive oil |
| Add | |
| 2 c | Shredded cabbage |

Sauté the cabbage until it wilts. Set aside in a bowl.
Add to the same skillet:

| 1 lb | Ground bison or beef |
|---|---|

Brown the meat. If it gets too dry, add:

| 2 T | Olive oil |
|---|---|
| Add | |
| 1 c | Mushrooms, sliced |
| 2 | Garlic cloves, minced and rested |
| ½ | Red onion, chopped |
| ¼ | Red pepper, deseeded, peeled and chopped |
| 1 T | Olive oil |

Cook until nicely browned. Put the cabbage back into
the skillet and stir well.

| Add | |
|---|---|
| 2 t | Chili powder |
| ¼ t | Oregano |
| 1 t | Cumin |
| 1 t | Salt |
| 1 t | Freshly ground black pepper |

Mix all the ingredients well. Sprinkle on top:

| ½ c | Shredded cheese |
|---|---|

Let cheese melt or place in the oven at 375° until cheese
melts, about 10 minutes.

Served with pickled beets and steamed broccoli.

# SWEET & SOUR BISON/BEEF MEATBALLS

### Goes well with mashed veggies | 15 minutes

|  | In a bowl, combine: |
|---|---|
| 1 lb | Ground bison or beef |
| 1 | Egg |
| 1 | Bread bun or thick slice of bread, crumbled in food processor |

Form into meatballs.

In a frying pan, heat oil:

| 1 T | Olive oil |
|---|---|

Fry meatballs to brown well all on all sides. Remove meatballs and set aside.

Add to the frying pan:

| 1 T | Olive oil |
|---|---|
| 1 | Large onion, chopped |

Sauté the onion until soft.

| Add |  |
|---|---|
| 2 T | Coconut sugar |
| 2 T | White vinegar (add enough vinegar to dissolve sugar) |
| 1 T | Mustard |

Stir well.

| Add |  |
|---|---|
| 2 c | *Katelyn's Tomato Sauce* |

Stir well. Add back the meatballs and spoon the sauce over them (add more tomato sauce if needed). Simmer for 15 minutes.

This pairs well with mashed sweet potato and root veggies.

# SWISS STEAK GB

| | |
|---|---|
| 2 | Chuck steaks (or 1 round steak) |

Cut the meat off the bone and remove any gristle.

For the marinade, combine:

| | |
|---|---|
| 2 T | Red wine or sherry |
| 1 T | Worcestershire sauce |
| ¼ c | Olive oil |

Put steak in a container and pour marinade over all its sides. Seal the container and place in the fridge for the day.

After its marinated, rinse the meat to reduce overspray. Place a cutting board in the sink and, one piece at a time, tenderize the meat with a meat hammer.

Sprinkle each piece with cassava flour and freshly ground black pepper. Use the meat hammer to infuse the meat. Repeat on the other side.

In a skillet, heat oil on medium-high:

| | |
|---|---|
| 2 T | Olive oil |

Add the meat and brown it well on both sides. Remove the meat.

Combine in the skillet:

| | |
|---|---|
| 2 | Medium onions, thinly sliced |
| 1 | Red pepper, deseeded, peeled and chopped |

Sauté, stirring frequently, until vegetables are brown.

Add
| | |
|---|---|
| 3 c | *Katelyn's Tomato Sauce* |
| 1 | Garlic clove, minced and rested |
| 1 t | Salt |
| ¼ t | Freshly ground black pepper |
| 1 | Bay leaf |

Stir well.

Add meat back in the pan. Simmer for a couple hours to continue to tenderize the meat.

Serve over mashed sweet potatoes with a side of *Mushrooms Sautéed* and beets or carrots.

Note: I chop and freeze leftover steak and sauce, and add it to beet borscht soup.

# Muffins

## MUFFINS ARE AN EXCELLENT ADDITION

Muffins are a delicious way to break-fast

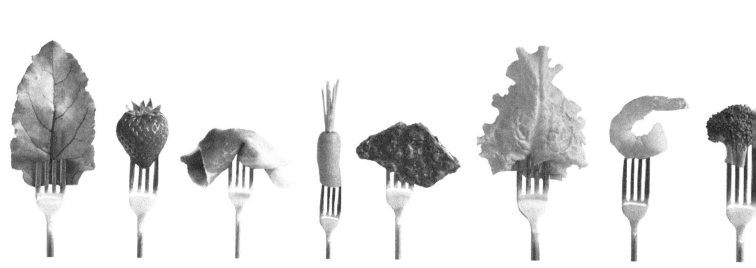

# APPLE CINNAMON MUFFINS

Makes 12 muffins

In a medium bowl, mix together:

| | |
|---|---|
| 1¼ c | Almond flour |
| 2 T | Tiger flour |
| 2 T | Flax meal |
| 2 T | Coconut flour |
| 1 t | Baking soda |
| ¼ t | Salt |
| 1 T | Cinnamon |
| 1 T | Ground ginger |
| 1/2 t | Allspice (heaping) |
| 1 packet | Stevia |

Set aside.

In a small bowl, mix together:

| | |
|---|---|
| 1 c | Apple, shredded with skins (one medium apple) |
| 1/2 c | Raisins (optional) |
| 2 | Eggs |
| 2 T | Maple syrup |
| ½ c | Coconut milk |
| 1 T | Coconut oil (MCT oil) |

Add wet ingredients to the dry and stir until blended.

Place 12 muffin parchment-paper liners in a muffin tin.
Fill with batter.

Bake at 350° for 25 minutes until golden brown.

# CARROT SPICE MUFFINS

Preheat oven 350° | Makes 12 muffins

In a large bowl, stir together:

| | |
|---|---|
| 1¼ c | Almond flour |
| ¼ c | Arrowroot flour |
| 2 T | Tiger nut flour |
| 2 T | Flax meal |
| 1 t | Baking soda |
| ½ t | Salt |
| 1½ t | Cinnamon |
| 1 t | Ground ginger |
| ¼ t | Nutmeg |
| 1 packet | Stevia |

In another bowl, mix together:

| | |
|---|---|
| ¼ c | Walnuts, chopped |
| 1 1/2 c | Carrots, grated (S-food processor works well for this) |

Fold carrots and walnuts into the dry ingredients.

In a small bowl, whisk together:

| | |
|---|---|
| 2 | Eggs, grass-pastured |
| ⅓ c | Avocado oil |
| ⅔ c | Coconut milk |
| 1 T | Yacon syrup |
| 2 T | Maple syrup |
| 2 t | Vanilla |

Add to the carrot-and-walnut mix. Stir until combined.

Place 12 muffin parchment-paper liners in a muffin tin.
Fill with batter.

Bake at 350° for 18 to 22 minutes, until toothpick comes out clean.

Note: Freeze for up to 3 months.

# CRANBERRY ORANGE MUFFINS

Preheat oven 350° | Makes 12 muffins

In a large bowl, mix together:

| | |
|---|---|
| 1½ c | Almond flour |
| ½ c | Cassava flour |
| ½ t | Baking soda |
| ¼ t | Salt |
| 1 packet | Stevia |

Stir well.

In a smaller bowl, add:

| | |
|---|---|
| 3 | Eggs |
| 4 T | Goat yogurt |
| 2 T | Yacon syrup |
| 1 T | Butter, melted |
| 1 T | Coconut oil, melted |

Whisk together until well blended.

Add wet ingredients to the dry, stirring well.

Fold in:

| | |
|---|---|
| ½ c | Cranberries |
| 1 T | Zest of an orange (heaping) |

Place 12 muffin parchment-paper liners in a muffin tin.
Fill with batter.

Bake at 350° for 20 to 22 minutes, until toothpick comes out clean.

Note: A nice variation - Zest of a lemon and 1T lemon juice

# Mushrooms

## MUSHROOMS ARE GUT BUDDY ESSENTIALS

Add as much variety as you can

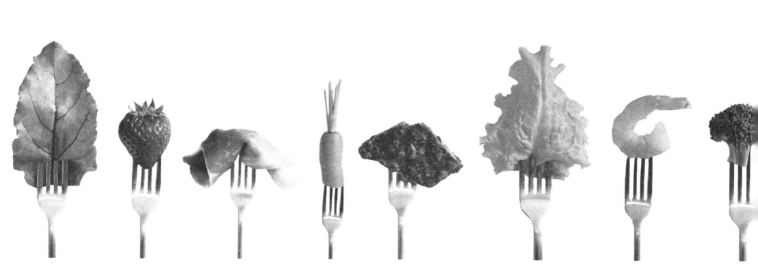

# MUSHROOM LENTIL STEW GB

|  | Turn an Instant Pot to "sauté" and cook: |
| --- | --- |
| 3 T | Olive oil |
| 2 c | Mushrooms, sliced |
|  | Cook until browned. |
| Add |  |
| ⅓ c | Red or green lentils (soaked in water 2 to 3 hours) |
|  | In a bowl, whisk together: |
| 2 T | Miso paste |
| ¼ c | Coconut amino |
|  | Add it to the Instant Pot along with: |
| 2 c | Kale, chopped |
| 3 | Green onions, chopped |
| 1½ c | Chicken or vegetable broth |

Turn the Instant Pot to "lentil" and add 10 minutes to cook. Let the steam release naturally.

Serve over mashed sweet potatoes with *Miso Baked Cod*.

# MUSHROOMS SAUTÉED GB

Serve as a side dish | 10 minutes

In a frying pan, heat oil on medium-high:

| | |
|---|---|
| 4 T | Olive oil |

Add

| | |
|---|---|
| 4 c | Mushrooms, chopped |
| 2 T | Onion, chopped |
| 1 T | Lemon juice |
| ½ t | Salt |
| To taste | Freshly ground black pepper |

Cook until the mushrooms are well browned, about 10 minutes.

Serve as a side dish.

# PORTOBELLO BURGERS GB

Delicious flavours

|  | Prepare your beans by soaking in water for 24 hours: |
| 4 c | Mixed dried beans (adzuki, black beans, pinto, etc.) |
|  | Rinse at least three times to decrease the lectin. |
|  | Add beans to an Instant Pot and combine with: |
| 6 c | Boiling water |
|  | Set the Instant Pot to 25 minutes. When it has completed its cycle, let the steam release naturally. |
|  | Drain the beans. There will be leftover beans for making refried beans. |
|  | In a large bowl, mash: |
| 2 c | Beans |

Add

| 2 c | Portobello mushrooms, chopped |
| 1 c | Broccoli, finely chopped |
| ½ c | Red onion, minced |
| 1 T | Worcestershire sauce |
| 1 t | Freshly ground black pepper |
| ¼ t | Dry mustard |
| ½ t | Dill seed or dill weed |
| ½ t | Celery seed |
| ½ t | Salt |
| 1 t | Minced garlic, rested |

|  | Mix well. |
|  | In a bowl, combine: |
| 3 | Eggs, beaten |
| 1 | Bread bun or thick slice of bread, crumbled in food processor |
| ¾ c | Parmesan cheese, grated |
|  | Add to mushroom mixture and mix well. Pat into burgers. |
|  | In a frying pan, heat oil: |
| 2 T | Olive oil |
|  | Cook burgers. If they don't stick together, add up to: |
| 2 T | Coconut flour |

# PORTOBELLO LOAF GB

Prepare your beans by soaking in water for 24 hours:

4 c    Mixed dried beans (adzuki, black beans, pinto, etc.)

Rinse at least three times to decrease the lectin.

Add beans to an Instant Pot and combine with:

6 c    Boiling water

Set the Instant Pot to 25 minutes. When it has completed its cycle, let the steam release naturally.

Drain the beans. There will be leftover beans for making refried beans.

In a large bowl, mash:

2 c    Beans

Add

2 c    Portobello mushrooms, chopped
1 c    Broccoli, finely chopped
½ c    Red onion, minced
1 T    Worcestershire sauce
1 t    Freshly ground black pepper
¼ t    Dry mustard
½ t    Dill seed or dill weed
½ t    Celery seed
½ t    Salt
1 t    Minced garlic, rested

Mix well.

In a bowl, combine:

3      Eggs, beaten
1      Bread bun, crumbled in food processor
¾ c    Parmesan cheese, grated

Grease a baking dish with:

1 T    Olive oil

Place the portobello mixture in the dish. Spread on top:

¾ c    *Katelyn's Tomato Sauce*

Sprinkle with final topping:

¾ c    Shredded cheddar cheese

Bake at 350° until the cheese is bubbling, about 20 minutes. Then increase temperature to 400° to brown the cheese.

Serve with *Katelyn's Brown Beans*, Caesar salad and pickles.

# Pasta

## MIRACLE NOODLES ARE FROM THE KONJAC ROOT

They are filling and high in viscous fiber

Yep, you read it right. Let's give Miracle Noodle pasta some special attention.

Be sure to buy the correct brand as some foods are calling themselves Miracle Noodle but add soy and other lectin items.

When you cut the bag of Miracle Noodle, it has a fishy smell. Follow the directions, which are simple. Rinse the noodles under running water and then boil the noodles. Next, pour off the water and dry-fry the noodles—they will not burn. Now they are ready for whatever recipe you want.

Miracle Noodle pasta is a delightful addition to any meal.

Reg even said, with our spaghetti and meatballs, he'd be hard-pressed to tell the difference from wheat noodles. The consistency is excellent.

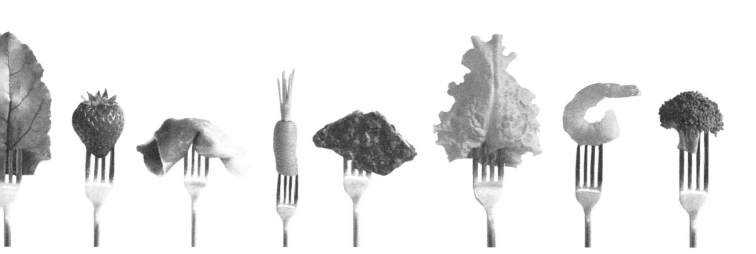

# FETTUCCINI ALFREDO GB

## Serve with roasted root veggies

Prepare Miracle Noodle pasta as directed and set aside.

In a pot, warm together:

| | |
|---|---|
| 2 T | Butter |
| 2 T | Olive oil |
| ¼ c | Parmesan cheese, shredded |
| 2 T | Goat yogurt |
| ¼ t | Salt |
| ⅛ t | Freshly ground black pepper |

Toss in the Miracle Noodle pasta and serve immediately.

# MAC & CHEESE WITH A TWIST GB

## Preheat oven 350° | Miracle Noodle

Prepare Miracle Noodle fettuccine as directed and set aside.

In a skillet, heat oil:

| | |
|---|---|
| 1 T | Olive oil |

Add
| | |
|---|---|
| 5 | Button mushrooms, thinly sliced |
| ½ | Medium red onion, chopped |

Sauté until nicely browned. Stir in:

| | |
|---|---|
| 2 | Slices prosciutto ham, chopped |

Place noodles in an 8" x 8" baking dish. Add the mushrooms, onions and prosciutto.

Add
| | |
|---|---|
| 1 c | Spinach or Swiss chard, chopped |

In a bowl, whisk together:

| | |
|---|---|
| 1½ c | Cheese, grated |
| ½ c | Coconut milk |
| 1 T | Butter or ghee |
| 1 | Egg, large |
| 1 t | Dijon mustard |
| 1 | Garlic clove, minced and rested |
| To taste | Salt and freshly ground black pepper |

Pour over the noodles.

Bake at 350° for 20 to 25 minutes until top has browned.

Serve with steamed veggies.

# MUSHROOM CHEESE NOODLES GB

## Great with steamed veggies and a salad

Prepare Miracle Noodle spaghetti as directed and set aside.

In a medium pan, sauté until nicely browned:

| | |
|---|---|
| 1 T | Butter |
| 1 T | Olive oil |
| ¾ c | Mushrooms, sliced |
| ½ c | Onions, chopped |

Add
| | |
|---|---|
| 1 t | Minced garlic, rested |
| To taste | Salt and freshly ground black pepper |

Cook for an additional few minutes.

Add prepared spaghetti noodles.

Add
| | |
|---|---|
| ¼ c | Parmesan cheese, grated |
| ¼ c | Cheddar cheese, grated |

Stir until mixed. Serve immediately.

Note: Certainly, this meal can accompany many of the meat dishes, but it also stands alone with some steamed root veggies and a salad.

# SWEET POTATO MAC & CHEESE GB

## Moist sage-spiced noodles

Prepare Miracle Noodle spinach pasta as directed and set aside.

In a pan, heat oil:

| | |
|---|---|
| 1 T | Olive oil |

Add
| | |
|---|---|
| 1 | Large sweet potato, peeled, chopped and steamed |
| 1 | Garlic clove, minced and rested |

Cook for a couple minutes.

Add
| | |
|---|---|
| 2 c | Kale, chopped (stems removed) or spinach |

Stir until slightly wilted.

In a large saucepan, heat:

| | |
|---|---|
| 1 T | Butter |

Add
| | |
|---|---|
| 1–2 T | Cassava flour |
| ⅛ t | Cayenne pepper |

Whisk in:

| | |
|---|---|
| 1½ c | Coconut milk |

Continue stirring until thickened.

Add sweet potato mixture.

Add
| | |
|---|---|
| 1 c | Cheddar cheese, shredded |
| 1 T | Dijon mustard |

Mix until smooth.

Place Miracle Noodle pasta in a baking dish. Pour cheese mixture overtop.

Top with sage breadcrumbs.

**Sage breadcrumbs**

In a bowl, combine:

| | |
|---|---|
| 1 | Bread bun, crumbled |
| 1 t | Sage |
| 1 T | Butter, melted |

Toss together.

# Pickles and Fermented Foods

## CREATE YOUR PRESERVES AT HOME

This really helps eliminate food additives

Pickling salt should be used in pickling and fermenting as there's no iodine or additives. Kosher salt can be substituted for pickling salt.

Here are directions for successful canning and preserving:

- Start with all clean utensils and jars
- Make sure jars are not cracked or chipped and both parts of lids are in good shape, with no dents or bending
- Always use very fresh, washed produce
- Precook the vegetables as directed on recipes—make sure food is still very hot just before canning
- Sterilize the jars for 10 minutes in boiling water and drop the lids in the pan to heat
- With pickles, be sure the brine is at a boiling point and pack jars as soon as you take them (one at a time) from the sterilizing container; seal immediately to be sure they're hot (pickles then don't need to be hot bath processed)
- For hot bath processing, make sure the jars are covered with water in the canner and start the timer once the water comes back to boiling
- Set a timer and leave the canner for the full length of time
- Retighten each jar as soon as it's taken out of the canner
- Do not tip the jars, especially tomato sauce
- If for some reason a jar doesn't seal, refrigerate and use it up soon; if a jar is not sealed after it's been in storage for a while, discard all the contents

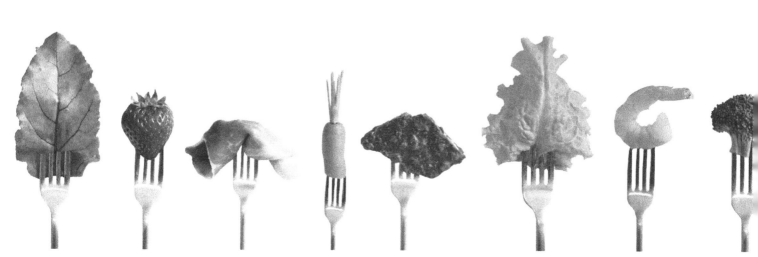

# DILL PICKLES

Crunchy pickles

In a pot, bring to a roiling boil:

| | |
|---|---|
| 1 qt | White vinegar |
| 3 qt | Water |
| ¼ c | Coarse pickling salt |

In each sterilized jar, pack to within ¾ inch from the top:

| | |
|---|---|
| | Pickling cucumbers |
| 2-3 | Garlic, peeled |
| 2 | Dill sprigs |

Pour boiling liquid into the hot jars to ¾ inch from the top.
Wipe the rims and placed hot lids on the jars, tightening well.

Makes about five jars of pickles.

Note: Try tasty variations—pickled carrots, kohlrabi, whole garlic, onions or beets.

# HOMEMADE HORSERADISH

Refrigerate or freeze

Start with horseradish root. Rinse off and use a vegetable brush to clean thoroughly. Peel enough root to equal:

| | |
|---|---|
| 1 c | Cubed horseradish |

Place it in a blender and add:

| | |
|---|---|
| 2 T | Water |
| ¾ c | White vinegar |
| 2 t | Coconut sugar |
| ¼ t | Salt |

Blend until smooth. Use a spatula to carefully transfer horseradish to a jar.

Warning: DO NOT SMELL as it will more than clean out your sinuses.

**Refrigerate:** Store in the fridge (it will keep for months) and shake jar well before using.

**Freeze:** Horseradish can be frozen in ice cube trays and then transferred to a freezer bag. An ice cube is about one tablespoon. Or place horseradish in a freezer bag, seal, and then flatten. When you want to use horseradish in a recipe, just break off as much as you want.

# REFRIGERATOR BEET PICKLES GB

## Keeps for months in refrigerator

In a large pot of water, place beetroot with enough water to cover them:

2 lb — Beets with 1 inch of stem

Bring water to boil and then reduce heat to medium-low. Cover and cook one hour or until beets are done.

Drain beets and let them cool enough to handle. Slip off the skins and cut into ¼-inch slices. Discard skins and stems.

Return beets to the pot.

Add
| | |
|---|---|
| ½ c | Red wine |
| ⅛ c | Balsamic vinegar |
| ⅛ c | Apple cider vinegar |
| ¼ c | Coconut sugar |
| ½ c | Water |
| ½ | Large shallot or red onion chopped |
| ¼ t | Pickling spice |

Add enough water to cover the beets. Bring to a boil then simmer for a few minutes. Cool and pack in a jar.

Place in your refrigerator. Let sit seven days before enjoying.

Note: These will keep for a number of months.

# REFRIGERATOR PICKLES

Crunchy

In a bowl, combine:

| | |
|---|---|
| 1 c | Coconut sugar |
| 1/2 c | White vinegar |
| 1/2 c | Apple cider vinegar |

Dissolve the sugar in the vinegar.

Add

| | |
|---|---|
| 8 c | Cucumbers, sliced |
| 1 T | Mustard seed |
| 1 c | Onion, thinly sliced |
| ¼ c | Pickling salt |
| 1 T | Celery seed |
| 2 | Green peppers, deseeded, peeled and cubed |
| 2 | Red peppers, deseeded, peeled and cubed |

Place in a large glass container with a lid and refrigerate.

Note: Store in the fridge for up to three months.

# SAUERKRAUT GB

## How-to

**Prepare cabbage**

Using fresh, organic cabbage (red, white or blend of both), fill a jar with:

| | |
|---|---|
| 1 medium | Cabbage, thinly shredded |

It should be enough to fill a jar that you can burp. Shred a bit more as the sauerkraut relaxes in the salt.

In a bowl, combine cabbage with:

| | |
|---|---|
| 1 T | Salt |

(This amount of salt is for a medium cabbage. Judge the salt based on the quantity you've shredded; too much salt can make your kraut tough.)

Work the cabbage with your hands to mix the salt in well and a brine starts to form.

**Fill the jar**

Add the cabbage to your jar, a few inches at a time, and pack down with a blunt instrument. This will activate more brine. Continue this process until you have filled the jar.

Place a layer of whole leaves on top and then add a weight. (Lee Valley Tools sells round glass weights that fit different jar sizes.)

Be sure all the cabbage remains submerged in the brine.

**Seal and age**

Close the lid and store at room temperature for 10 to 14 days or until the brine quits bubbling. The sauerkraut is complete when the brine reabsorbs.

**Keep checking**

Open the jar every day to burp the off gasses. It will have a pungent smell, which is normal.

If any mould appears, remove it and be sure the cabbage is in the brine.

When the sauerkraut is ready, remove the large leaves and discard.

**Store**

Store the sauerkraut in the fridge and enjoy every day.

# Poultry

## LOOK FOR GRASS- OR HAY-FED POULTRY

### Free-range

Using poultry that's been grass- or hay-fed (instead of soy-, corn- or grain-fed) can help reduce the lectins in your chicken meals. When chickens are in the pasture, they forage for grubs and bugs, which are really good for them. The meat may be a bit different because the chickens actually get exercise.

Grass-finished meat is especially crucial for those of us who are super sensitive to lectins in food.

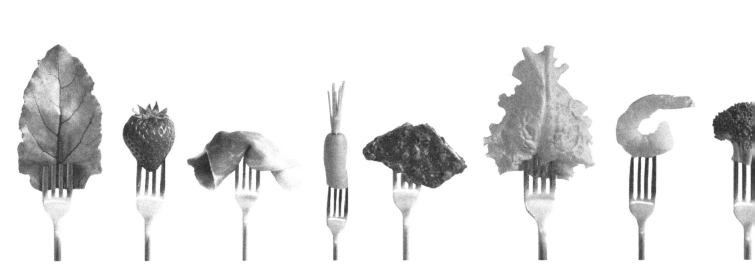

# ASIAN NOODLE BOWL GB

## Quick, filling meal

Prepare Miracle Noodle angel hair pasta as directed and set aside.

In a large pot, combine:

| | |
|---|---|
| 1 | Chicken breast, butterfly cut, then cut in cubes (or use leftover chicken) |
| 3 T | Coconut amino |
| 1 T | Ginger, minced |
| 1 | Garlic clove, minced and rested |
| 2 T | Rice wine vinegar |
| 2 T | Toasted sesame oil |

Start heating on medium-high.

| | |
|---|---|
| Add | |
| 4 c | Chicken broth (if using homemade, add salt to taste) |

Cook to boiling. When chicken is cooked through, add Miracle Noodle pasta.

| | |
|---|---|
| Add | |
| 2 c | Broccoli chunks |
| ¼ c | Red pepper, thinly sliced(deseeded and peeled ) |
| 1 | Small carrot, grated |

Cook until broccoli turns bright green.

| | |
|---|---|
| Add | |
| 4 | Green onions, sliced |

In the bottom of large soup bowls, place:

| | |
|---|---|
| 1 c | Spinach in each bowl |

Pour the chicken noodle broth over the spinach. Serve immediately.

# CHICKEN BALSAMIC VEGETABLE BAKE

Preheat oven 375° | Marinate 20 minutes

In a small bowl, combine:

| | |
|---|---|
| ¼ c | Balsamic vinegar |
| 2 T | Olive or avocado oil |
| 3 | Garlic cloves, minced and rested |
| 1 T | Basil |
| 1 t | Thyme |
| ½ t | Salt |
| ¼ t | Freshly ground black pepper |

Stir well.

Add

2       Small chicken breasts

Toss the chicken with the herb blend. Marinate in fridge for 20 minutes.

In a baking dish, combine:

| | |
|---|---|
| ½ | Broccoli head, chopped |
| 1 | Kohlrabi, peeled and sliced into slim sticks |
| 2 | Carrots, peeled and sliced into slim sticks |
| 1 c | Mushrooms, sliced |
| 1 | Small red onion, sliced |

Mix together. Drizzle with half the marinade liquid.

Place the chicken on the vegetable bed. Drizzle the remaining liquid over the chicken and vegetables.

Bake at 375° for 25 minutes until the chicken has cooked thoroughly.

# CHICKEN BREAST & PESTO BAKE

Preheat oven 375° | 8–10 minutes

In a bowl, toss together:

| | |
|---|---|
| 1 | Chicken breast, cut butterfly style |
| ¼–½ c | *Pesto Sauce* |

Place chicken in a baking dish. Top chicken with any remaining pesto. Bake at 375° for 8 to 10 minutes depending on the thickness of the chicken breast.

Serve with baked sweet potato rounds and a garden salad.

# CHICKEN BREAST STUFFED

Preheat oven 350° | 35 minutes

Steam until wilted:

| | |
|---|---|
| 2 c | Spinach |

Place in a bowl.

Add

| | |
|---|---|
| 3 T | Goat yogurt |
| 1 c | Shredded cheddar cheese |
| 1 t | Parsley |
| ¼ t | Thyme |
| ¼ t | Oregano |
| ¼ t | Basil |
| ¼ t | Rosemary |
| 1 | Garlic clove, minced and rested |
| To taste | Salt and freshly ground black pepper |

Mix well. Divide mixture into two and press into:

| | |
|---|---|
| 2 | Chicken breasts, ¾ butterfly cut and slightly flattened |

Use toothpicks to close. Place in baking dish.

Bake at 350° for 35 minutes until well done.

# CHICKEN BROCCOLI BAKE

## Preheat oven 400°

|       | In an oven-safe skillet, heat oil on medium-high: |
|-------|---|
| 2 T   | Olive oil |
| Add   | |
| 1     | Chicken breast, cut this into two butterfly pieces |
|       | Cook chicken until nicely browned on all sides. Push chicken aside and add to skillet: |
| 1     | Garlic clove, finely chopped and rested |
| ½     | Large onion, chopped |
|       | Cook until the onion is wilted and browned. |
| Add   | |
| ½     | Broccoli head, cut in chunks, with broccoli stems peeled and sliced |
|       | Whisk into the onions and garlic: |
| ½ c   | Chicken broth (or leftover vegetable water) |
|       | Put a lid on the skillet and let the broccoli turn a bright green. Combine with the chicken and broccoli in the skillet: |
| ¼ t   | Thyme |
| ¼ t   | Oregano |
| ½ t   | Parsley |
|       | Top with: |
| ½ c   | Parmesan cheese, grated |
| ½ c   | Cheddar cheese, shredded |
|       | Bake at 400° until cheese is bubbling and browns slightly. |

# CHICKEN CACCIATORE

Instant Pot | Serve with Miracle Noodle

|       | In an Instant Pot, add: |
|-------|-------------------------|
| 1 T   | Olive oil |
| 4     | Chicken thighs |

Set Instant Pot on "sauté" and cook chicken pieces on all sides.

| Add   |                        |
|-------|------------------------|
| 2     | Medium onions, chopped |
| 1     | Large red pepper, cut into strips |

Continue to sauté.

| Add   |                        |
|-------|------------------------|
| 8     | Medium Roma tomatoes, quartered |
| ¾ c   | *Katelyn's Tomato Sauce* |
| ½ c   | Red wine |
| 2 t   | Minced garlic, rested |
| ¾ t   | Basil |
| ¼ t   | Freshly ground black pepper |

Set Instant Pot to "meat" and then add 10 minutes. Cook and let the steam release naturally.

When the pressure releases, open the lid and stir in to thicken slightly:

| 1 T   | Cassava flour |
|-------|---------------|

Serve with Miracle Noodle fettuccine, and steamed cauliflower and carrots.

Note: Instant Pot destroys lectins, so there is no need to deseed and peel the red pepper.

# CHICKEN IN ROSEMARY MUSHROOM CREAM GB

## Serve with sweet potatoes

|  | In a skillet, heat oil on medium-high: |
|---|---|
| 1 T | Olive oil |

Add
| 4 | Chicken thighs |
| To taste | Salt and freshly ground black pepper |

Brown the chicken heat until cooked, stirring as needed.
Remove chicken to a dish.

In the skillet:

Add
| 1 c | Mushrooms, chopped |
| 3 | Garlic cloves, minced and rested |

Sauté mushrooms until browned.

Add
| ½ c | Chicken broth |
| 1 T | Balsamic vinegar |
| 2 t | Rosemary |
| 1 T | Parsley |

Bring to boil and then turn skillet down to medium-low.

Add
| ½ c | Goat yogurt |
| ¼ c | Parmesan cheese, grated |

Stir until well blended, stirring all the brown bits around
the pan.

Add
| To taste | Salt and freshly ground black pepper |

Place chicken thighs back in the skillet and reheat thoroughly.

Serve with mashed sweet potatoes, beets and Brussels sprouts.

# CHICKEN PARMIGIANA GB

|  | In a frying pan, heat oil: |
|---|---|
| 1½ T | Olive oil |

Add
| 1 c | Mushrooms, chopped |
| ½ c | Cilantro, chopped |
| ½ c | Onions, chopped |
| 2 | Garlic cloves, minced and rested |

Sauté for 5 minutes.

Add
| ½ t | Basil |
| ½ t | Oregano |
| 3 T | *Katelyn's Tomato Sauce* |

Cook for 5 more minutes.

In a baking dish, arrange:

| 4 | Chicken thighs |

Pour the vegetables over the chicken and top with:

| ½ c | Shredded mozzarella cheese |
| ½ c | Grated parmesan cheese |

Bake at 425° for 25 to 30 minutes until chicken is thoroughly cooked.

# CHICKEN PICCATA

|       | Prepare chicken by flattening with a meat hammer: |
|-------|---------------------------------------------------|
| 1     | Large chicken breast, butterfly cut and cut in two |
|       | In a shallow dish (such as a pie plate), add: |
| 1 T   | Cassava flour |

Dredge chicken breasts in flour on one side and use the meat hammer to infuse. Flip over and repeat on the other side.

In a heated skillet on medium-high:

Add
| 1 T   | Olive oil |
|-------|-----------|
| 1 T   | Butter |

Add chicken, brown it on both sides and remove to a plate.

In the skillet:

Add
| ½ c   | White wine |
|-------|------------|
| ¼ c   | Lemon juice |
| 2 T   | Capers |
| 2     | Garlic cloves, minced and rested |

Scrape the pan to release any chicken bits and brown oils.

Bring to a boil and add the chicken back to the pan. Cook for 2 minutes, allowing the sauce to thicken a bit.

Serve with a garden salad and a variety of root veggies.

# CHICKEN/TURKEY POT PIE FILLING

|  | In a skillet, heat oil on medium-high: |
| 2 T | Olive oil |

Add
| 1 | Yellow onion, chopped |
| 4 | Medium carrots, diced |
| 2 | Celery stalks, chopped |
| 1 | Medium sweet potato, cut in small cubes |

Cook the vegetables until done, about 5 minutes.

Add
| 2 c | Chicken or turkey, cubed cooked (use leftovers) |
| 3 t | Cassava flour |
| 1 c | Chicken broth |
| 1 t | Dried thyme |
| ½ t | Dried rosemary |
| To taste | Salt and freshly ground black pepper |
| 2 T | Olive oil |

Bring to a simmer, allowing to thicken, and then remove from the heat.

Note: If too dry, add more chicken broth.

Divide the filling into four oven-proof single-serving containers, like ramekins or onion soup bowls.

Cover with *Grain-Free Pie Dough* and prick with a fork.

# CHICKEN WITH MUSHROOMS, TOMATOES & PARMESAN GB

In an Instant Pot, combine:

| | |
|---|---|
| 4 | Chicken thighs |
| 1 T | Olive oil |

Turn Instant Pot to "sauté" and brown chicken on both sides.

Add
| | |
|---|---|
| 1 c | Mushrooms, sliced |
| 1 c | Onion, chopped |
| 2 | Garlic cloves, minced and rested |
| ½ | Red pepper, thinly sliced |
| 1 t | Thyme |
| 1 t | Sage |
| ½ c | Red wine |
| ¼ c | Chicken broth |
| 8 | Roma tomatoes (can be frozen) |
| 1 c | *Katelyn's Tomato Sauce* |
| 1 | Parmesan rind |

Set the pressure cooker on "meat" and add 10 minutes. Let it cook and let the pressure release naturally.

Note: This pairs nicely with *Celeriac/Cauliflower Mashed* and steamed beets or beet pickles.

# CHICKEN WHOLE WITH VEGGIES

Instant Pot

|  | Turn Instant Pot to "sauté" and heat oil: |
|---|---|
| 3 T | Olive oil |
| Add | |
| 1 | Whole chicken |
|  | Sauté well on all sides and then place breast-side up. |
| Add | |
| 1 | Onion, chopped |
| 3 | Garlic cloves, minced and rested |
| 1 | Large sweet potato, quartered |
| 3 | Large carrots, whole |
| 1 t | Salt |
| 1 T | Parsley |
| ½ t | Thyme |
| ½ t | Basil |
| ½ c | Chicken broth (or water) |

Turn the Instant Pot to "chicken" and then add time to equal 45 minutes. Put the top on.

Let it pressure up and then release naturally.

Note: Whole daikon radishes (approximately 1 cup) add a wonderful flavour.

# CHICKEN STRIPS BREADED

Place in a food processor:

| | |
|---|---|
| ½ c | Almonds, sliced |
| ½ | Bread bun, crumbled |
| Pinch | Cayenne pepper |
| ½ t | Ginger |
| 1 t | Paprika |
| 1 t | Oregano |
| ½ t | Thyme |
| 1 t | Parsley |
| ½ t | Salt |

Blend until fine and then place on a shallow plate.

In a shallow bowl, beat:

| | |
|---|---|
| 1 | Egg |

Grease a baking dish:

| | |
|---|---|
| 1 T | Olive oil |

Prepare the chicken pieces:

| | |
|---|---|
| 1 | Chicken breast, butterflied and sliced into long wide strips |

A few strips at a time, dip the chicken into the egg and then drop the pieces into the breaded mixture to coat.

Place each coated piece into the baking dish. Once all pieces are coated and in the baking dish, drizzle olive oil on the top.

Bake at 375° for 15 to 20 minutes (depending on thickness of the breast) until chicken is cooked thoroughly.

**Dipping sauce**

In a blender, combine:

| | |
|---|---|
| 5 | Dates, pitted and steeped 1 hour in small amount of water |
| 2 T | Dijon mustard |

Mix well.

# CHICKEN STRIPS IN COCONUT

## Preheat oven 375° | 12–20 minutes

|  |  |
|---|---|
|  | In a shallow bowl, place: |
| 2 T | Coconut flour |
|  | In another shallow bowl, place: |
| 1 | Egg, beaten |
|  | In a third shallow bowl, place: |
| ¼ c | Coconut bits |
| 2 t | Flax seed, milled |
| ½ t | Garlic, minced and rested |
| ½ t | Onion, minced |
| ¼ t | Paprika |
| ⅛ t | Cayenne pepper |
| To taste | Salt and freshly ground black pepper |
|  | Prepare the chicken: |
| 1 | Chicken breast, butterflied and cut into 1-inch strips |

Dip the chicken strips, one at a time, into the flour and then the egg, and then the seasonings. Place them in an oiled baking dish and drizzle with olive oil. Sprinkle any remaining seasonings on top and bake at 375° for 12 to 20 minutes or until chicken is thoroughly cooked.

**Curry dip**

|  |  |
|---|---|
|  | In a bowl, combine: |
| ¼ c | Goat yogurt |
| ¼ c | Avocado mayonnaise |
| 2 t | Curry powder |
| ¼ t | Hot sauce |

Chill and serve with the chicken strips.

# CHICKEN WITH TERIYAKI VEGETABLES

## Serve over cauliflower rice

|  | Prepare the chicken: |
|---|---|
| 1 | Chicken breast, butterflied and cut into ½-inch-long strips |

In a small bowl, combine:

| 3 T | Sherry or red wine |
|---|---|
| ½ T | Coconut sugar |
| 2 T | Water |
| 3 T | Coconut amino (soy replacement) |
| 2 T | Olive oil |
| 1½ t | Ground ginger |

Whisk all together. Add the chicken and marinate 15 to 30 minutes.

Prepare the vegetables:

| 1 t | Garlic clove, minced and rested |
|---|---|
| ½ | Red pepper, deseeded, peeled and cut into long strips |
| 1 | Large carrot, cut into 2½-inch chunks and then into thin strips |

In a frying pan, heat oil on medium-high:

| 1 T | Olive oil |
|---|---|

Add the chicken and marinade, and stir fry until chicken is cooked thoroughly, at least 2 minutes.

Add the vegetables and sauté for another 2 minutes.

Serve over cauliflower rice.

# CHINESE CHICKEN FRIED RICE

## One-dish meal

|     | In a small bowl, whisk together: |
|-----|-----|
| 1   | Egg |
| 1 T | Water |

In a frying pan on medium-high heat:

| Add |  |
|-----|-----|
| 1 T | Butter |
| 1 T | Olive oil |

Add the egg and cook it. Remove from pan and slice into thin strips. Set aside.

In the frying pan:

| Add |  |
|-----|-----|
| 1   | Onion, chopped |

Sauté until soft.

| Add |  |
|-----|-----|
| 2 c | Cauliflower rice |
| 2 T | Coconut amino |
| 1 t | Freshly ground black pepper |
| 1 c | Chicken meat, cooked and chopped |

Stir together about 5 minutes. Stir the egg back in and serve.

# CUBED CHICKEN & MUSHROOMS
# IN RED WINE GB

### Served with mashed cauliflower

|  | Pan sear in a skillet: |
|---|---|
| 1 T | Olive oil |
| 1 | Chicken breast, cubed |

Cook until done. Push chicken to the side of the skillet.

Add
| 2 c | Mushrooms, sliced |
| 1 T | Olive oil |

Cook until nice and brown. Push mushrooms to the side.

Add
| 2 T | Shallots, chopped |

Cook for a few minutes.

Add
| ¼ c | Red wine |

Simmer lightly. Stir in:

| ½ c | Goat yogurt |
| To taste | Salt and freshly ground black pepper |

Then stir in:

| ¼ c | Cauliflower vegetable juice (from the cooked vegetables below) |

Stir in to thicken:

| 1 T | Cassava flour |

Serve with *Celeriac/Cauliflower Mashed*, daikon sprouts and pickles.

# CURRY CHICKEN & PEARS

Served with root veggies

|  |  |
|---|---|
|  | In a frying pan, heat oil: |
| 2 T | Olive oil |
| Add |  |
| 1 | Chicken breast, butterflied and cut in two |
|  | Brown well on both sides. |
| Add |  |
| ½ T | Lime zest |
| ½ T | Ginger, minced |
| ½ c | Chicken stock |
| 1 | Bay leaf |
| ½ | Red pepper, deseeded, peeled and sliced into strips |
| ½ c | Coconut milk |
| 2 | Large garlic cloves, minced and rested |
| 1 | Green onion, diagonally sliced |
| 3 T | Coconut amino |
| ½ t | Cinnamon |
| 1 t | Curry |
| ½ | Pear, thinly sliced |
| 1 | Generous grind of black pepper |
|  | Bring to a boil. |
|  | Stir in to thicken: |
| 2 T | Cassava flour |
|  | Turn low to simmer. |
|  | Serve with roasted parsnips and carrots. |

# HONEY TURMERIC CHICKEN

In a bowl, mix together:

| | |
|---|---|
| 2 | Garlic cloves, minced and rested |
| 1½ T | Maple syrup |
| 1 T | Coconut aminos |
| ¾ t | Turmeric powder |
| Pinch | Cayenne pepper |
| ¼ | Salt |
| 2 T | Olive oil |

Add

| | |
|---|---|
| 2 | Chicken breasts |

Stir well. Place everything in a baking dish.

Drizzle with:

| | |
|---|---|
| 1 T | Olive oil |

Cook for 20 minutes until the chicken is well done.

# MIRACLE RICE FRIED CHICKEN WITH MUSHROOMS GB

## Miracle Noodle

| | |
|---|---|
| | Prepare Miracle Noodle rice noodles as directed and set aside. |
| | In a large pan, heat oil on medium-high: |
| 2 t | Sesame oil |
| Add | |
| 2 | Green onions, chopped |
| ¾ c | Mushrooms, chopped |
| 2 c | Broccoli, chopped |
| | Stir fry for a couple of minutes. Move the vegetables to the side. Heat in the pan: |
| 1 T | Olive oil |
| Add | |
| 1 | Egg, slightly beaten |
| | Scramble the egg. |
| Add | |
| 1 | Chicken breast, finely chopped |
| | Stir together with the vegetables and heat together. Add the Miracle Noodle rice noodles along with: |
| 2 T | Coconut amino |
| | Stir all together to warm, and then serve. |

# NELL'S THAI CHICKEN

## Chicken with a yummy dressing

|        | In a frying pan, heat oil:                             |
|--------|--------------------------------------------------------|
| 2 T    | Olive oil                                              |
| Add    |                                                        |
| 1      | Chicken breast, butterflied and cut into 1-inch strips |
|        | Brown nicely on both sides.                            |
| Add    |                                                        |
| 1      | Red pepper, deseeded, peeled and cut into strips       |
| 2 T    | Coconut amino                                          |
| 1 T    | Sherry                                                 |
|        | Sauté together until red pepper is just wilting.       |

**Dressing**

|       | In a small bowl, whisk together: |
|-------|----------------------------------|
| 1 T   | Lime juice                       |
| 2 t   | Coconut sugar                    |
| 2 t   | Almond butter                    |
| 2 t   | Coconut amino                    |
| 2 T   | Olive oil                        |

Pour dressing over chicken.

Serve with cauliflower rice and steamed broccoli.

# ROASTED ROSEMARY CHICKEN

Preheat oven 325° | Cook for 3 hours

| | |
|---|---|
| 3–4 lb | Whole chicken |
| | Stuff the cavity with: |
| 5 | Garlic cloves, peeled |
| 4 | Fresh rosemary sprigs |
| 1 | Orange with its peel, cut into 6 to 8 pieces |
| | In a small bowl, combine: |
| 1 | Fresh rosemary sprig, chopped |
| 2 T | Olive oil |
| 2 T | Orange zest |
| 1 T | Lemon zest |
| 1 T | Coconut sugar |

Mix well and spread over the breasts and limbs of the chicken.

Bake at 325° for 3 hours until internal temperature reaches 195°.

Serve with salad and roasted carrots.

# TURKEY À LA KING GB

<hr>

## Great use of leftover turkey

<hr>

|        | In a frying pan, heat: |
|--------|------------------------|
| 6 T | Butter or ghee |

Add
| 4 c | Mushrooms, sliced |
| ¼ c | Peppers, thinly sliced |

Sauté the vegetables.

Add
| 3 c | Cooked turkey, diced (use leftovers) |

Cook until warm. Stir in:

| 6 T | Cassava flour |

Slowly and gradually, add:

| 1 c | Chicken broth |
| 2 c | Goat yogurt |

Stirring the sauce constantly until it thickens, reduce to low and cook for 5 minutes.

In a cup, place:

| 2 | Egg yolks |

Stir in a tablespoon of the hot liquid. Gradually stir that into the turkey mixture, stirring rapidly to prevent lumps.

Stir in:

| 1 (4 oz) jar | Pimentos, drained |
| 2 T | Sherry or red wine |
| 1 t | Salt |

Let this mixture cook for a couple of minutes.

Serve immediately over toasted bread buns.

# Salads

## OUR GUT BUDDIES LOVES SALAD

Eat your greens

When you bring your greens home:

- Cut or break them into bite-size pieces
- Wash them in a salad spinner
- Store them in food-cloth bag or repurposed containers for sealing

It makes for very fast table presentation.

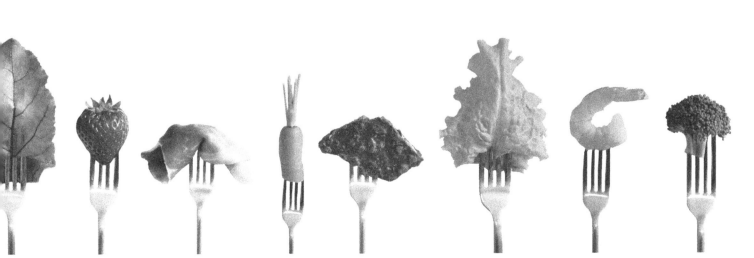

# BEETS SHREDDED WITH WALNUTS & KALE GB

Nice side salad

In a large bowl, combine:

| | |
|---|---|
| 3 | Medium raw beets, shredded |
| 2 c | Kale, chopped or Swiss chard, stems removed |
| ½ c | Walnuts, chopped |
| ½ c | Raisins |

Toss together.

**Dressing**

In a small bowl, combine:

| | |
|---|---|
| 1 T | Lemon juice |
| 2 T | Olive oil |
| 2 t | Red wine vinegar |
| 1 t | Dijon mustard |

Toss together.

Toss with salad ingredients and serve.

# BROCCOLI CAULIFLOWER APPLE SALAD

## Crisp salad

Lightly steam:

| | |
|---|---|
| 2 c | Broccoli, chopped |
| 2 c | Cauliflower, chopped |

Set aside in a large bowl to cool.

Add
| | |
|---|---|
| 1 | Apple, cored and chopped |
| ½ | Medium red onion, chopped |
| ¼ c | Walnuts, chopped |
| ¼ c | Raisins |
| 1 | Medium carrot, shredded |

**Dressing**

Blend together:

| | |
|---|---|
| ½ c | Goat yogurt |
| ¼ c | Avocado mayonnaise |
| 1 T | Balsamic vinegar |
| 1 T | Maple syrup |

Toss with salad ingredients and serve.

# BROCCOLI CAULIFLOWER SALAD

## Quick side vegetable salad

In a large bowl, combine:

| | |
|---|---|
| ½ | Broccoli head, finely chopped |
| ½ | Small cauliflower head, finely chopped |
| 1 | Red onion, chopped |
| ½ c | Raisins, rinsed, or dried cranberries |

**Dressing**

In a small bowl, combine:

| | |
|---|---|
| ½ c | Avocado mayonnaise |
| ½ c | Goat yogurt |
| 1 T | Apple cider vinegar |
| 2 T | Coconut milk |
| 3 T | Balsamic vinegar |

Stir together.

Toss with salad ingredients and serve.

# COLESLAW

## Refreshing side salad

In a food processor, shred:

| | |
|---|---|
| ½ | Medium red or green cabbage (or ¼ of each) |
| 1½ | Green peppers, deseeded, peeled and thinly chopped |
| 1 | Carrot, grated |
| 1 | Celery stalk, thinly chopped |
| 2 T | Red onion, minced |
| 2 T | Raisins or cranberries |

Toss together and add *Coleslaw Dressing*.

# CUCUMBER SALAD

Crunchy

In a medium bowl, combine:

| | |
|---|---|
| 2 | Medium cucumbers, peeled, deseeded and sliced |
| 1 | Large red onion, thinly sliced |

**Dressing**

In a small bowl, whisk together:

| | |
|---|---|
| ¼ c | Apple cider vinegar |
| 2 T | Olive oil |
| ¼ t | Freshly ground black pepper |
| ¼ t | Salt |
| 1 t | Dill weed |
| 1 T | Maple syrup |

Pour the dressing over the salad and mix well.

# GREEN SALAD WITH BEETS & RED ONION

Fruity garden salad

In a large bowl, combine:

| | |
|---|---|
| 4 c | Mixed salad greens |
| 2 | Small beets, sliced |
| ½ c | Red onion, thinly sliced |
| ¼ c | Blueberries |
| ¼ c | Walnuts, chopped |
| ¼ c | Feta cheese, crumbled |
| ¼ t | Oregano |

Toss and serve with *Raspberry/Blackberry Dressing* or *Balsamic Vinaigrette Dressing*.

# MAYO-LESS SLAW

### Zesty salad

In a large bowl, combine:

| | |
|---|---|
| 3 c | Green or red cabbage, shredded |
| 1 | Large carrot, shredded |
| 4 | Green onions, sliced |

**Dressing**

In a small bowl, whisk together:

| | |
|---|---|
| 4 T | Olive oil |
| 4 T | Balsamic vinegar |
| 1 t | Lemon zest |
| 2 | Garlic cloves, minced and rested |
| 1 T | Parsley |
| ½ t | Basil |
| ½ t | Thyme |
| To taste | Salt and freshly ground black pepper |

Pour over vegetables, toss well and refrigerate until ready to serve.

# NUTTY KOHLRABI SLAW

### Refreshing Spicy Salad

In a bowl, combine:

| | |
|---|---|
| ¼ c | Goat yogurt |
| 1 T | Dijon mustard |
| 1 T | Balsamic vinegar |
| 2 t | Horseradish |
| 1 | Garlic clove, minced and rested |
| 1 t | Capers |
| ¼ t | Salt |
| ¼ t | Freshly ground black pepper |
| 1 | Purple kohlrabi, shredded |
| ¼ c | Chopped walnuts |
| ½ c | Daikon radish sprouts |

Stir and refrigerate.

# SPICY CAESAR CHICKEN SALAD

## Caesar Salad with a Twist

In a large bowl, combine:

| | |
|---|---|
| ½ | Chicken breast, cooked and chopped (use leftovers) |
| 2 | Green onions, chopped |
| ½ | Red pepper, deseeded, peeled and chopped |
| 1 | Celery stalk, finely chopped |
| 3 c | Romaine lettuce, chopped |

Toss together.

Serve with *Spicy Salad Dressing*.

# SPINACH PEAR SALAD

## Delightful

In a large bowl:

Add
| | |
|---|---|
| 4 c | Spinach (washed) |
| 1 | Pear, cored and thinly sliced (in season) |
| ½ c | Cranberries |
| ¼ c | Walnuts, toasted |
| ¼ c | Red onion, thinly sliced |

**Dressing**

In a small bowl, whisk together:

| | |
|---|---|
| 1½ T | Olive oil |
| 1 T | Red wine vinegar |
| ¼ t | Salt |
| ¼ t | Freshly ground black pepper |

Toss with salad ingredients.

Add
| | |
|---|---|
| To taste | Salt and freshly ground black pepper |

Serve.

# Sauces

## SAUCES ADD THE DELICIOUS FLAVOUR

A variety of flavours add to the enjoyment to your meals

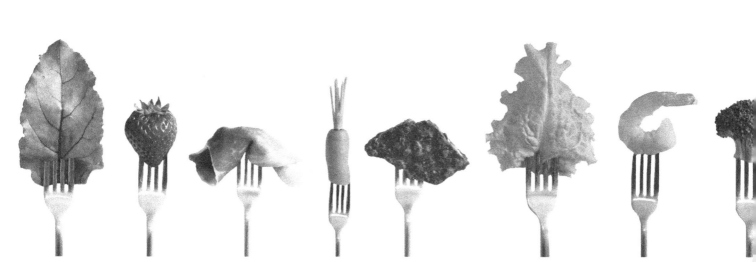

# CHICKEN STRIPS DIPPING SAUCE

## Chicken sauce

Soak for one hour in a small amount of water:

| | |
|---|---|
| 5 | Dates, pitted |
| Add | |
| 2 T | Dijon mustard |

Blend well and serve.


# CILANTRO PESTO

## Freeze for up to 3 months

In a blender, combine:

| | |
|---|---|
| 1 c | Cilantro, packed |
| ½ c | Almonds, sliced |
| 3 | Large garlic cloves |

Puree until smooth.

| | |
|---|---|
| Add | |
| ¼ c | Parmesan cheese, grated |
| ½ c | Olive oil |
| ½ t | Salt |

Puree into a smooth paste.

Pesto can be frozen in ice cube trays then popped out into freezer bags.

Note: Keeps in freezer for up to three months.

# CURRY DIP FOR CHICKEN

Delicious

In a small bowl, combine:

| | |
|---|---|
| ¼ c | Goat yogurt |
| ¼ c | Avocado mayonnaise |
| 2 t | Curry powder |
| ¼ t | Hot sauce |

Chill and serve.

# KATELYN'S TOMATO SAUCE

## Pressure cooker

Place in a pressure cooker:

|       | Tomatoes, chopped |
|-------|-------------------|
| 2     | Red peppers, chopped |
|       | Hot peppers (to taste), chopped |
| ½ c   | Water |

The food should reach the fill line. Pressure cook for 20 minutes.

In a food processor, chop vegetables:

|   |                      |
|---|----------------------|
| 3 | Medium carrots       |
| 3 | Medium celery stalks |
| 6 | Garlic cloves        |
| 2 | Large onions         |

Chop vegetables, a bit at a time. Then place them in a very large 8-quart pot along with:

| 3 T | Olive oil |
|-----|-----------|

Sauté until vegetables are nice and soft.

Add
| 2 T | Parsley |
|-----|---------|
| 1 T | Pickling salt |
| 2 T | Paprika |
| 1 T | Balsamic vinegar |
| 2 T | Oregano |
| 2 T | Basil |
| 2 T | Thyme |
| 2 T | Olive oil |

When the tomatoes and peppers have finished cooking in the pressure cooker, add them to the large pot.

Bring everything to a boil and then reduce the heat. Simmer until it starts to thicken. (Depending on how much liquid is in the sauce, this can take hours.)

Using an immersion blender, blend the vegetables until you reach a thickened tomato sauce consistency. Continue to simmer, stirring occasionally until the tomato sauce reaches your desired thickness.

Pour contents into sterilized quart jars and seal with sterilized lids.

Place the jars in a canner for a hot water bath (with the water covering the jars).

Boil for 20 minutes. (If using pint jars, boil for 10 minutes in a boiling water bath.)

Check that all the jars and tops are in good shape. Wipe the rim of the jar before sealing.

When processing is complete, remove the jars and place (without tipping) onto a cutting board to allow to cool.

The lids will pop as each jar seals. Do not touch the lids during this process.

Store tomato sauce jars in a cool, dark place for up to a year.

Note: Be sure to date the jars.

# MUSHROOM SAUCE GB

## Great topping for meat

|  | In a pan, heat oil: |
| --- | --- |
| 2 T | Olive oil |
| Add | |
| 1½ c | Mushrooms, sliced |
| ½ t | Salt |
|  | Sauté until mushrooms are nice and brown. |
| Add | |
| 2 T | Cassava flour |
|  | Stir well, allowing the flour to combine gradually. |
| Add | |
| ½ c | Chicken broth |
|  | Stir well. |
| Add | |
| ¼ c | Goat yogurt |
| ½ t | Dijon mustard |
| 1 T | Sherry |
|  | Stir well. |

Note: This sauce is excellent for chicken, bison, beef or pork; it pairs well with broccoli salad and beets.

# MUSTARD SAUCE

### Topping for chicken, beef or shrimp

In a small bowl, combine:

| | |
|---|---|
| ¼ c | Avocado mayo |
| ½ | Avocado, mashed |
| 1 | Garlic clove, minced and rested |
| 1 T | Dry mustard |
| ¼ t | *Sriracha Sauce* |
| Dash | Worcestershire sauce |

Stir ingredients together well.

Note: Excellent with chicken strips, beef and shrimp.


# PESTO SAUCE

### Pasta sauce

In a food processor, process:

| | |
|---|---|
| ½ c | Spinach |
| ½ c | Kale, chopped or Swiss chard, stems removed |

| | |
|---|---|
| Add | |
| ½ c | Almonds, shaved |
| ¼ c | Olive oil |
| 2 T | Water |
| ¼ t | Salt |
| 2 | Garlic cloves |
| | Juice of a lemon |

Process until a nice thick consistency.

Place the pesto sauce in ice cube trays. When frozen, pop them out into a freezer bag. The cubes can keep for three months.

I have used basil, parsley or any combination together.

Note: Prepare it early, and reheat to use with Miracle Noodle pasta.

# SHRIMP COCKTAIL SAUCE

Excellent dipping sauce for shrimp

In a bowl, combine:

| | |
|---|---|
| 1 c | *Katelyn's Tomato Sauce* |
| 1–2 T | Horseradish (to taste) |
| 1 T | Lemon juice |
| ½ t | Worcestershire sauce |
| To taste | Salt and freshly ground pepper |

Stir well. Place in a jar and refrigerate.

Note: This sauce will keep for a few weeks in the refrigerator.

# SHRIMP SAUCE

Quick and easy

In a small pot, combine:

| | |
|---|---|
| ¼ c | Parsley, chopped |
| 6 | Garlic cloves, minced and rested |
| | Juice of half a lemon |
| 2 T | Olive oil |
| 2 T | Butter |
| To taste | Salt and freshly ground black pepper |

Stir and melt together.

Serve warm over grilled shrimp.

# SRIRACHA SAUCE GB

Fermented

In a blender, add:

| | |
|---|---|
| 1 lb | Jalapeños peppers, stems removed, chopped |
| ½ lb | Red chili peppers, stems removed, chopped |
| 6 | Garlic cloves, chopped |
| 1 T | Maple syrup |
| 1 packet | Stevia |
| 1 T | Salt |
| 5 T | Water |

Blend until smooth.

Place the sauce in a glass jar, cover with a lid and put in a cool, dark place. Stir every day, scraping down the sides until it starts to ferment and bubble.

Pour the fermented mixture in the blender.

Add

| | |
|---|---|
| ¾ c | White vinegar |
| 2 T | Balsamic vinegar |

Blend well.

Using a strainer, strain into a pot, pushing through as much pulp as possible. Discard the remaining seeds and skins.

Bring to a boil, stirring often, and then reduce the heat. Let it simmer until the sauce thickens, 5 to 10 minutes.

Let the sauce cool to room temperature. Pour it into a glass jar and store in the fridge with the date on the lid.

The sauce will keep for up to six months.

Note: Wear gloves when handling the peppers. If you get pepper juice on your skin, be sure to have some real lemons to squeeze for the juice to neutralize the acidity. Because this is fermented, it is allowed with the Plant Paradox eating.

# TANGY THAI SAUCE

## Delicious over grilled chicken or fish

In a pot, combine:

| | |
|---|---|
| ½ c | Apple cider vinegar |
| ¼ c | Coconut sugar |
| 4 | Garlic cloves, minced and rested |
| ⅛ t | Chili powder |
| ⅛ t | Cayenne pepper |
| 2 T | Coconut amino |

Bring to a boil and then reduce to medium-low heat, stirring occasionally. Allow the liquid to reduce.

When the sauce has thickened a bit, cool it and place it in a jar.

Note: The sauce will keep for up to three weeks in the refrigerator.

# TARTAR SAUCE

## Great with fish

In a jar, combine:

| | |
|---|---|
| ⅓ c | Avocado mayonnaise |
| ½ | Large dill pickle, finely chopped |
| ½ t | Dill weed |
| 1 t | Lemon juice |
| 2 T | Green onion, chopped |
| To taste | Freshly ground black pepper |

Mix well and refrigerate.

Note: Use within a week.

# Seafood and Fish

## EAT FISH 2 OR 3 TIMES A WEEK

### Just don't overdo it

It's important to consume fish 2 or 3 times a week for omega-3. Big fish types have an increased risk of mercury in their flesh, so you should limit your consumption.

Some examples of big fish types are halibut, tuna, swordfish and mackerel. Choose instead, salmon, anchovies, sardines, cod, trout, clams, snapper and shrimp.

Purchasing wild seafood will reduce your intake of lectins and toxic substances found in farmed fish. But, take note: research shows fish in the marketplace is often mislabelled and not what it says it is.

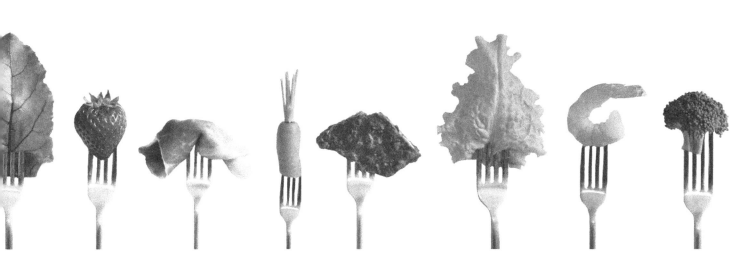

# BAKED SALMON/COD IN MISO SAUCE GB

Preheat oven 350° | 15–30 minutes

|      | In a baking dish, place: |
|------|---------------------------|
| 2    | Wild salmon or cod steaks |
|      | In a bowl, whisk together: |
| 2 T  | Miso paste |
| 4 T  | Coconut amino |
| 4 T  | Chicken broth |

Pour half over the fish, turn the fish over and top with remaining sauce.

Bake at 350° until the fish flakes easily. This can be 15 to 30 minutes, depending on the thickness of the fish.

# BAKED SALMON IN MUSTARD SAUCE

Preheat oven 375° | 20–30 minutes

In a baking dish, arrange a bed of vegetables:

Carrots, cut into thin sticks
Red pepper, deseeded, peeled and sliced lengthways
Red onion, sliced
Garlic clove, chopped

Drizzle with:

| | |
|---|---|
| 2 T | Olive oil |
| To taste | Salt and pepper |

Toss to coat the vegetables nicely.

Place in the baking dish on top of the bed of vegetables:

| | |
|---|---|
| 8–12 oz | Wild salmon |

In a small bowl, whisk together:

| | |
|---|---|
| 3 T | Dried parsley |
| 2 T | Dijon mustard |
| | Juice of a lemon |
| 2 T | Olive oil |
| 2 t | Minced garlic, rested |

Drizzle on the fish and vegetables.

Bake at 375° until the fish flakes and vegetables are done, about 20 to 30 minutes.

# BAKED TROUT

|          | In a piece of tin foil, place: |
|----------|--------------------------------|
| 1        | Trout                          |

|          | In a bowl, combine:                         |
|----------|---------------------------------------------|
| 2 T      | Lemon juice                                 |
| 2        | Garlic cloves, minced and rested            |
| 3 T      | Melted butter                               |
| To taste | Salt                                        |
| ¼ t      | Oregano                                     |
| ¼        | Red pepper, deseeded, peeled and chopped    |

Mix well. Pour over the trout and seal the tin foil. Bake at 375° for 20 to 25 minutes.

Check doneness in the centre, and then broil for 2 to 3 minutes.

Sprinkle with parsley and serve.

# BREADED SALMON WITH LEMON GARLIC HERBS

Preheat oven 400° | 8–12 minutes

|  | In a small bowl, whisk together: |
|---|---|
| 1 T | Ghee |
| 1 T | Melted butter |
|  | Juice of a lemon |
|  | Zest of a lemon |
| 1 T | Parsley |
| 1 t | Dill weed (chopped if using frozen) |
| 1 | Garlic clove, minced and rested |
| To taste | Salt and freshly ground black pepper |

Set aside.

In a food processor, crumble:

| 1 | Bread bun or thick slice of bread |
|---|---|

Pat dry:

| 8–12 oz | Salmon or cod |
|---|---|

Coat the fish with half the breadcrumbs and place in a baking dish.

Pour the liquid over the breaded fish and then sprinkle the remaining breadcrumbs overtop.

Sprinkle on top:

| ¼ c | Parmesan cheese |
|---|---|

Bake at 400° for 8 to 12 minutes until the fish flakes nicely.

# COD WITH LEMON, PARMESAN & GARLIC

---

Preheat oven 350° | 12–15 minutes

---

In a small bowl, combine:

|  | Juice of a lemon |
|---|---|
|  | Zest of half a lemon |
| 1 T | Parsley |
| 1 t | Dill weed |
| 2 | Garlic cloves, minced and rested |
| 3 T | Butter, melted or ghee |
| ¾ c | Grated parmesan |

Mix well.

In a baking dish, place:

| 12 oz | Wild cod |
|---|---|

Cover with the liquid mix. Bake at 350° until the cod flakes, about 12 to 15 minutes.


Note: This recipe works well with salmon or red snapper.

# COD WITH STEWED PORTOBELLOS & ONIONS GB

## Preheat oven 350°

|          | In a large skillet, heat oil:                                    |
|----------|------------------------------------------------------------------|
| 2 T      | Olive oil                                                        |
| Add      |                                                                  |
| 2 t      | Fresh rosemary                                                   |
| ½        | Red onion, very thinly sliced                                    |
| 1        | Large portobello mushroom, chopped                               |
| 2        | Garlic cloves, minced and rested                                 |

Cook the vegetables over medium-high heat until nicely browned, stirring frequently.

| Add       |                                      |
|-----------|--------------------------------------|
| 8–10 oz   | Wild cod                             |
| 2 T       | Olive oil                            |
| To taste  | Salt and freshly ground black pepper |

Transfer to a baking dish and bake at 350° until fish flakes easily.

Serve with carrots and parsnips mashed together with 1 tablespoon butter and fresh Daikon radish sprouts.

# FISH & CHIPS

Preheat oven 400° | Serve with sweet potato fries

Preheat air fryer for five minutes and oil the pan before battered fish is added.

**Batter**

In a bowl, whisk together:

| | |
|---|---|
| ⅜ c | Tapioca flour |
| ⅛ c | Coconut flour |
| ½ t | Salt |

In a small bowl, whisk together:

| | |
|---|---|
| 1 | Large egg |
| ⅛ c | Sparkling water (Pellegrino) |

Blend the wet ingredients with the dry ingredients.

Pat dry:

| | |
|---|---|
| 10 oz | Wild cod |

Dip the cod in the batter, and then place it in the air fryer.

Drizzle with and remaining batter and:

| | |
|---|---|
| 1 T | Olive oil |

Bake at 400° until cod is flaky, about 12 to 15 minutes, depending on the thickness of the cod.

The air dryer makes the cod batter nice and crisp. Drizzle olive oil on the cod.

Serve with oven-baked yam fries or *Sweet Potato Fries*.

Serve with *Tartar Sauce*, *Coleslaw* or a nice spring salad; these complement fish and chips nicely.

# FISH CAKES

## Serve with salad

In a bowl, mash with a fork:

6–8 oz         Cooked fish (use leftovers or 1 small can wild salmon)

If there is leftover breading from the fish, throw that into a food processor, crumble and add it to the bowl.

Add
1 c         Sweet potato, mashed
¼         Red onion, chopped
1         Celery stalk, chopped (or minced in a food processor)
1         Egg

Stir well.

Add
1 T         Parsley
½ t         Salt
½ t         Freshly ground black pepper
2 T         Coconut flour

Form into 5 patties. Let them rest on a plate.

In a skillet, heat oil on medium-high:

2 T         Coconut oil

Place the fish cakes in the frying pan and cook for 3 to 4 minutes on each side. Reduce the heat and continue to cook for an additional 3 to 4 minutes. The cakes are ready when browned well.

Serve with a Caesar or garden salad, fresh sprouts and *Refrigerator Beet Pickles*.

# GREEK PRAWNS IN TOMATO SAUCE

## Italian flare

|  | In a medium pan, heat oil: |
|---|---|
| 2 T | Olive oil |
| Add | |
| 10–12 | Shrimp |
| 1½ c | Mushrooms, sliced |
| 2 | Garlic cloves, minced and rested |
|  | Cook until the shrimp and mushrooms are browned. |
| Add | |
| ½ c | White or red wine |
| ¾ c | *Katelyn's Tomato Sauce* |
| 1 T | Balsamic vinegar |
|  | Simmer to combine the flavours. |
| Add | |
| ¼ c | Feta cheese, crumbled |
|  | Serve when the feta has melted. |
|  | Serve with Miracle Noodle fettuccine and root veggies. |

# PESTO FISH CAKES

In a food processor, crumble:

1 Bread bun or thick bread slice

In a bowl, combine breadcrumbs with:

| | |
|---|---|
| 2 c | Cooked fish (use leftovers) |
| ¼ c | Pesto |
| 1 | Small onion, finely diced |
| 1 | Egg |
| 1 T | Lemon zest |
| 1 T | Goat yogurt |
| 1 T | Coconut flour |

Form into patties and place in the fridge for 15 minutes.

Heat the grill and coat with oil:

2 T Coconut oil

Cook the fish cakes for 3 to 4 minutes, and then flip and cook the other side. Reduce the heat to low and cook for an additional 3 minutes.

Serve with *Tartar Sauce*, *Sriracha Sauce* and a garden salad.

# ROASTED SALMON & VEGGIES

---
### Preheat oven 350°
---

|  |  |
|---|---|
|  | In a baking dish, layer: |
| 2 c | Asparagus spears or broccoli, chopped |
| 1 | Red onion, thinly sliced |
| 1 | Medium sweet potato, sliced into ½-inch slices |
|  | In a small bowl, combine: |
| ¼ c | Coconut amino |
| ¼ c | Balsamic vinegar |
| ¼ c | Avocado oil |
| 2 | Garlic cloves, minced and rested |

Pour half the liquid over the vegetables.

Add
1          Wild salmon fillet

Pour the remaining sauce over the salmon.

Bake at 350° until the salmon flakes easily and the vegetables have cooked.

# SALMON AVOCADO WRAPS

---
### A nice change for lunch
---

|  |  |
|---|---|
|  | In a bowl, mix together: |
| ¼ c | Parmesan cheese, grated |
| ¼ c | Celery, minced |
| 1 | Green onion, finely chopped |
| ½ | Avocado, mashed |
|  | Juice of half a lime |
| 1 can | Wild salmon, drained |
| 1 T | Avocado mayo |
| To taste | Salt and freshly ground black pepper |

Chill until ready.

Place a handful of lettuce on a flax meal tortilla and spoon a third of the mixture on top. Roll and grill, if you choose.

Note: For a variation, add a dressing, *Sriracha Sauce* or *Homemade Horseradish*.

# SALMON/COD IN MAPLE BALSAMIC

Preheat oven 400° | Quick and easy

|        |                                                   |
|--------|---------------------------------------------------|
|        | Grease a baking dish with oil:                    |
| 1 T    | Olive oil                                         |
| Add    |                                                   |
| 2      | Salmon or cod pieces                              |
|        | In a small bowl, whisk together:                  |
| ¼ t    | Salt                                              |
| ¼ t    | Freshly ground black pepper                       |
| ⅛ c    | Balsamic vinegar                                  |
| 2 T    | Maple balsamic vinegar                            |
| 2 T    | Olive oil                                         |
| 2 T    | Shallot, minced                                   |

Pour over the fish, turning the fish once to coat well.

Bake at 400° for 10 to 15 minutes.

# SHRIMP GRILLED WITH PEARS

## Grill at 400° | Made in minutes

|          |                                        |
|----------|----------------------------------------|
|          | Soak for 30 minutes in water:          |
| 8        | Large jumbo shrimp                     |
|          | Drain and toss with:                   |
| 1 T      | Olive oil                              |
| 1 t      | Basil                                  |
| 1 t      | Oregano                                |
| To taste | Salt and freshly ground pepper         |

Skewer shrimp and place in an air fryer. Grill at 400° for about
4 to 6 minutes depending on the size of the shrimp.

In a large bowl, whisk together:

| 1 T | Rice vinegar |
|-----|--------------|
| 1 T | Lime juice   |
| 1 t | Lime zest    |
| 1 T | Maple syrup  |
| 1 T | Olive oil    |

| Add |                                  |
|-----|----------------------------------|
| ½   | Pear, quartered, cored and chopped |
| ½   | Medium red onion, chopped        |
| 2 T | Parsley                          |

Stir to mix.

On a plate, pour the fruit onion mixture equally over the shrimp skewers.

Serve with steamed carrots and a salad.

# SNAPPER, COD OR SALMON PARMIGIANA

Preheat oven 425° | Tomato and cheese taste

|         | In a frying pan, heat oil: |
|---------|----------------------------|
| 1½ T    | Olive oil                  |

Add
| 1 c   | Mushrooms, chopped            |
|-------|-------------------------------|
| ½ c   | Cilantro or parsley, chopped  |
| ½ c   | Onion, chopped                |
| 2     | Garlic cloves, minced and rested |

Sauté for 5 minutes until vegetables are nice and soft.

Add
| ½ t   | Basil                   |
|-------|-------------------------|
| ½ t   | Oregano                 |
| 3 T   | *Katelyn's Tomato Sauce* |

Cook for 2 to 3 minutes on medium heat.

Place the fish in a baking dish and pour the vegetables on top.

Top with:
| ½ c   | Mozzarella, shredded |
|-------|----------------------|
| ½ c   | Parmesan, grated     |

Bake at 425° for 10 to 15 minutes until the fish flakes with a fork.

# SHRIMP MUSHROOMS WITH NOODLES GB

An Asian Flair

Prepare Miracle Noodle spinach spaghetti as directed and set aside.

In a large skillet, heat oil on medium-high:

| | |
|---|---|
| 1 T | Olive oil |

Add

| | |
|---|---|
| 8–12 | Shrimp |

Cook and stir the shrimp for 3 to 4 minutes and then remove from the skillet.

Add to the skillet:

| | |
|---|---|
| 1 T | Butter |
| 2 T | Olive oil |
| 1 T | Sesame oil |
| 2 c | Mushrooms, sliced |
| 2 | Garlic cloves, minced and rested |
| 1 c | Red onion, sliced |
| ¼ c | Red pepper, chopped (deseeded and peeled) |

Cook until vegetables are wilted and browning slightly.

In a small bowl, combine:

| | |
|---|---|
| ½ c | Red wine |
| ¼ c | Coconut amino (soy replacement) |
| 1 T | Coconut sugar |
| 3 T | Water |
| 2 | Green onions, sliced |
| To taste | Salt and freshly ground black pepper |

Return the shrimp back to the skillet and pour the liquid overtop.

Cook until boiling and then turn the heat off.

Serve over the Miracle Noodle spinach pasta.

# ZESTY SHRIMP WITH PESTO NOODLES

Interesting twist

Prepare Miracle Noodle pasta as directed and set aside.

**Pesto sauce**

In a processor, add:

| | |
|---|---|
| ½ c | Spinach, chopped |
| ½ c | Kale, chopped or Swiss chard, stems removed |
| ½ c | Almonds, shaved |
| ¼ c | Olive oil |
| 2 T | Water |
| ¼ t | Salt |
| 2 | Garlic cloves |
| | Juice of a lemon |

Process until a nice thick consistency. Add to the
Miracle Noodle pasta.

In a large skillet, heat on medium-high:

| | |
|---|---|
| 1 T | Olive oil |
| 1 t | Butter |

Add
| | |
|---|---|
| 8–10 | Jumbo shrimp |
| 1 t | Chili powder |
| 1 t | Cumin |
| 1 t | Minced garlic, rested |
| To taste | Salt and freshly ground black pepper |

Add the shrimp and seasonings and stir to gently coat all the shrimp.

Cook for about 3 minutes. Serve immediately over the pesto noodles.

# Seasonings, Spices and Marinades

## LEARN TO USE A VARIETY OF SPICES

Spice up your meals

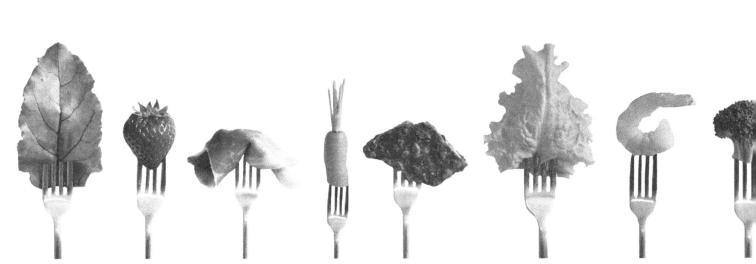

# HOMEMADE SHAKE & BAKE

## Keep frozen until needed

In a bowl, combine:

| | |
|---|---|
| 3 c | Bread buns, crumbled |
| 1 T | Salt |
| 1 T | Celery seed |
| 3 t | Paprika |
| 1 t | Coconut sugar |
| 1 t | Freshly ground black pepper |
| 1 t | Dried garlic |
| ½ t | Cayenne pepper |
| ½ t | Parsley |
| ½ t | Basil |
| ½ t | Oregano |
| ¼ t | Thyme |

Place in a freezer bag and freeze. Use as needed.

# LEMON/LIME PEPPER

## Shaker spice

Prepare the lemon/lime rinds.

6      Juiced lemon or lime rinds (or a combination)

Cut the rinds into small chunks and dehydrate until crispy.

In a bowl, combine equal parts:

Dehydrated lemon/lime rinds
Black peppercorns
Celeriac or celery seeds

Blend to a powder.

Add
1 t      Sea salt

Blend and add to a shaker for the kitchen table.

# MEAT MARINADE

### Marinate all day

In a bowl, whisk together:

| | |
|---|---|
| ½ c | Red wine |
| 1 T | Olive oil |
| 2–3 | Garlic cloves, minced and rested |
| ½ t | Rosemary |
| ½ t | Basil |
| ½ t | Oregano |
| 2 T | *Katelyn's Tomato Sauce* |
| 1 T | Apple cider vinegar |
| 1 t | Worcestershire sauce |

To use, pour over meat, coating evenly, and place in a sealed container in the fridge for the day.

# MEAT TENDERIZER/MARINADE

### Marinate all day

In a bowl, combine:

| | |
|---|---|
| 2 T | Red wine or sherry |
| 1 T | Worcestershire sauce |
| ¼ c | Olive oil |

To use, pour over a steak, coating evenly, and place in a sealed container in the fridge for the day.

# Snacks and Appetizers

## SOCIAL EVENT LIFE SAVERS

Here is something for everyone

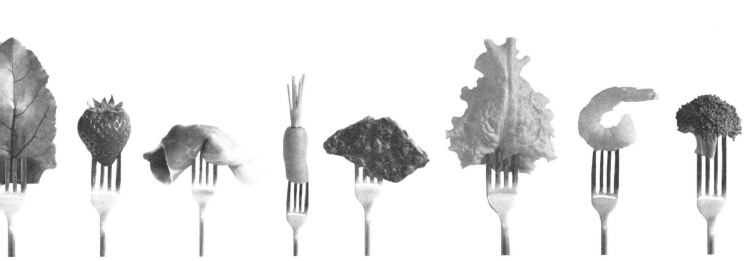

# CHICKEN WING SNACKS

Preheat oven 425° | Marinate 15–30 minutes

In a blender, combine:

| | |
|---|---|
| 2 T | Toasted sesame oil |
| ½ c | Coconut amino |
| ¼ c | Sherry |
| ¼ c | *Katelyn's Tomato Sauce* |
| 1 T | Ginger, minced |
| ½ t | Freshly ground black pepper |

Blend and then pour over:

| | |
|---|---|
| 12 | Chicken wings |

Place wings in the fridge and marinate for 15 to 30 minutes.

Place wings with marinade in a flat pan. Bake at 425° for about 30 to 40 minutes (turning wings over halfway) until nicely browned.

Toss with:

| | |
|---|---|
| 3 | Green onions, sliced |

Serve warm or cold.

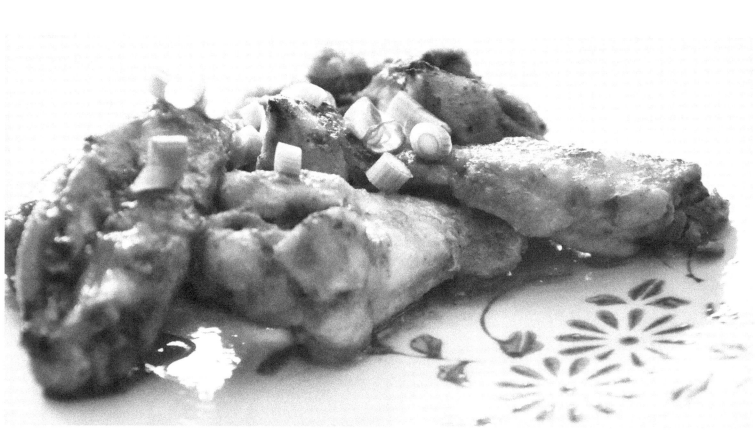

# COCONUT NUT BAR GB

Preheat oven 350° | 20 minutes

In a food processor, add:

| | |
|---|---|
| 1½ c | Sliced almonds |
| ½ c | Pecans,chopped |
| ½ c | Walnuts,chopped |
| ¼ c | Coconut bits |
| 2 T | Cacao nibs |
| 2 t | Cinnamon |
| Dash | Salt |

Process until nuts are chunky.

In a large bowl, combine:

| | |
|---|---|
| ¼ c | Coconut oil, melted |
| 4 T | Almond butter |
| 1 t | Vanilla |
| 2 T | Maple syrup |
| 3 | Eggs |

Blend well until the ingredients are thoroughly combined. Add the nut chunks and mix well.

Place in a greased 8" x 10" baking dish. Bake at 350° for 20 minutes until golden brown.

In a pan, melt:

| | |
|---|---|
| ¼ c | 80% dark chocolate pieces |

Add

| | |
|---|---|
| ⅛ c | Coconut bits |

Drizzle the melted mixture overtop the baked bars.

Cool and then cut into squares.

# ITALIAN CRACKERS

In a medium-sized bowl, combine:

| | |
|---|---|
| 1½ c | Almond flour |
| ½ c | Cassava flour |
| ½ t | Baking powder |
| 1 T | Parsley |
| 1 t | Oregano |
| 1 t | Sage |
| 1 t | Thyme |
| 1 t | Rosemary |
| 2 T | Flax meal |
| ½ t | Salt |

With the back of a tablespoon, press down on the almond flour to break up any lumps. Mix well.

Add
| | |
|---|---|
| 1 T | Olive oil |
| ½ c | Cold water |

Stir together until evenly moist.

Place on a greased baking stone, and press somewhat flat. Cover with parchment paper and roll out to a similar thickness all over, covering as much of the pan as possible (take your time).

Score the dough into equal-sized crackers, using a pizza cutter. (I use a pastry cutter from Lee Valley tools. I wet the cutters and rinse a few times as the dough will start to stick on the cutter).

Bake at 350° for 24 minutes. Then take the browned crackers off the edges and bake for another 10 minutes. Repeat twice more, each time removing the edge crackers and baking another 10 minutes. Use a thin metal flipper upside down to help release the crackers from the baking stone.

Hint: Place a rubber band under the baking stone as you roll out the dough. It will stop the stone from sliding away from you.

# STUFFED MUSHROOMS GB

## Great appetizer

|  | On a large grill at medium-high heat, arrange mushrooms stem-side up: |
|---|---|
| 20 | Small brown or white mushrooms, stems removed |
|  | Cook for 5 minutes, moving the mushrooms occasionally. Turn the mushrooms over and cook for another 5 minutes. Place the mushrooms on a paper towel stem-side down and let cool. |

**Stuffing**

|  | The stuffing can be made beforehand and refrigerated. |
|---|---|
|  | In a blender, place: |
| 4 T | Almonds, shaved and toasted |
| ¼ | Red pepper, deseeded and peeled |
| 1 c | Parsley |
| 1 c | Cilantro |
| ½ c | Parmesan cheese, grated |
|  | Zest of half a lime |
|  | Juice of a lime |
| ¼ t | Salt |
| 1 | Garlic clove, chopped |
|  | Blend until everything is chopped. |
|  | As the blender is running slowly drizzle in: |
| 2 T | Olive oil |
|  | Blend well. |
|  | Fill each mushroom cap with 1 teaspoon of filling and top evenly with either parmesan cheese or more toasted sliced almonds. |

Hint: Freeze the mushroom stems for use in other recipes such as *Mushroom Soup* or *Veggie-Stuffed Mushrooms*.

# SWEET & SALTY TRAIL MIX

Preheat oven 375° | 18 minutes

In a bowl, toss together:

| | |
|---|---|
| 1 c | Almonds |
| 1 c | Pecans |
| ½ c | Walnuts |
| ¼ c | Hemp seed |

Add
| | |
|---|---|
| 3 T | Maple syrup |
| ½ t | Celery salt |
| ¼ t | Sea salt |
| ½ t | Cumin |
| ¼ t | Cinnamon |

Toss together well.

Line a baking dish with parchment paper. Place the mix in the baking dish and bake at 375° for 18 minutes, until the nuts are toasted. Stir while the mixture is still warm.

Add
| | |
|---|---|
| ½ c | Cranberries or raisins |

Let trail mix cool then store in sealed bags and place in the fridge.

# VEGGIE-STUFFED MUSHROOMS GB

Preheat oven 375° | 20–25 minutes

|           | In a frying pan, heat oil on medium-high: |
|-----------|-------------------------------------------|
| 1 T       | Olive oil                                 |

Add
| 10  | Mushroom stems, chopped small   |
| 1   | Onion, finely chopped           |
| 2   | Garlic cloves, minced and rested |
| 1 c | Fresh parsley, chopped          |

Cook until nicely browned.

Add
| 2 c | Spinach, chopped |

Cook until wilted and then place in a bowl.

Add
| 1         | Bread bun, crumbled                     |
| ¼ c       | Feta cheese, crumbled                   |
| ¼ c       | Parmesan cheese, grated                 |
| To taste  | Salt and freshly ground black pepper    |

Mix all together to form the stuffing and then stuff:

| 10 | Large mushrooms |

Arrange on a baking tray and bake at 375° for 20 to 25 minutes.

Note: This works also without the bread bun.

# Soups

## SAVE YOUR LEFTOVER VEGETABLE WATER

### Makes great soup stock

Here are a few hints for making soup:

- When steaming or boiling vegetables never throw out the leftover water
- Let the vegetable water cool a bit and then pour it into a glass jar
- Let cool to room temperature and then place it in a freezer container
- Keep adding broth to the frozen broth until the freezer container is filled
- It becomes awesome soup stock

Be sure to cool soups to room temperature before you put them
in a freezer container. Plastic containers should not be heated and
should be allowed to thaw at room temperature.

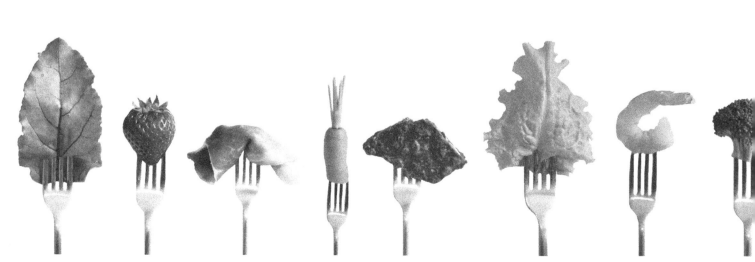

# ASPARAGUS SOUP

Immersion blender

|        | In a frying pan, heat: |
|--------|------------------------|
| 1 T    | Olive oil |
| 1 T    | Butter |
| Add    | |
| 4 c    | Asparagus stem ends (add full asparagus if needed to fill out quantity) |
| 2 t    | Lemon |
| 1 t    | Lemon zest |

Sauté until stems have softened.

Gradually add while slowly stirring:

| 2 T    | Cassava flour |

Once well stirred, add:

| ½ c    | Goat yogurt |
| 1 c    | Leftover vegetable broth or water |
| 1 T    | Parsley |
| Add    | |
| ½ t    | Salt and freshly ground black pepper |

Using an immersion blender, blend to a creamy consistency.

Serve with chopped chives.

# BEET BORSCHT BISON SOUP GB

## Instant Pot

In an Instant Pot, place:

| | |
|---|---|
| 2 T | Olive oil |
| 1 | Large yellow or red onion, chopped |
| ¼ | Red pepper, deseeded and diced |
| 2 | Small sweet potatoes, diced |
| 2 | Large carrots, chopped |
| 2 | Celery stalks, diced |

Turn the Instant Pot to "sauté" and cook the vegetables until soft.

| | |
|---|---|
| Add | |
| 5 | Garlic cloves, minced and rested |
| ½ t | Dill weed |
| 2½ c | Beets, peeled and cubed |
| 6 c | Red or green cabbage, chopped |
| 2 | Bay leaves |
| 1½ t | Salt |
| 1 t | Freshly ground black pepper |
| ½ jar | *Katelyn's Tomato Sauce* |
| 1 L | Chicken broth |
| 4 T | Red wine vinegar |
| ¼ lb | Bison steak, cooked and chopped (use leftovers) |

Turn the Instant Pot to "soup" and then add 15 minutes.
Let it cook and release the steam naturally.

Note: You can make this vegetarian by omitting the bison steak.

Hint: It tastes even better after freezing.

# BLACK BEAN SOUP GB

Instant Pot

|       | In an Instant Pot, combine: |
|-------|------------------------------|
| 2 T   | Olive oil |
| 2 c   | Onions, chopped |
| 2 c   | Carrots, chopped |
| 4     | Garlic cloves, minced and rested |

Turn Instant Pot to "sauté" and cook the vegetables until well softened.

|       | Add |
|-------|-----|
| 4 c   | Black beans (2 cups dried beans soaked 12 hours and rinsed well) |
| 1 L   | Chicken broth |
| ½ t   | Coconut sugar |
| 1 t   | Cumin |
| 2 T   | Parsley, dried |

Cover and pressure cook for 25 minutes.

Using an immersion blender, puree the soup.

Serve with:

| 1 T | Goat yogurt |
| 1T  | Parsley |

# CAULIFLOWER BROCCOLI SWEET POTATO SOUP

Instant Pot

|  | In an Instant Pot, heat oil: |
| --- | --- |
| 1 T | Olive oil |
| Add | |
| 1 c | Onion, chopped |
| 2 | Garlic cloves, minced and rested |

Turn the Instant Pot to "sauté" and cook the vegetables.

| Add | |
| --- | --- |
| 1 | Red pepper, deseeded and chopped |
| 1 | Medium cauliflower, chopped |
| 1 | Medium broccoli, chopped |
| 2 | Small sweet potatoes, chopped |
| 1 L | Chicken broth (Kirkland organic chicken broth is wheat-free) |

Turn the Instant Pot to "soup" and add 10 minutes. Let the pressure release naturally.

Using an immersion blender, blend soup to a creamy consistency.

Sprinkle with:

| ⅛ c | Cheddar cheese, shredded |
| --- | --- |
| 1 t | Chives, chopped (per bowl) |

Serve.

# CHICKEN BONE BROTH GB

In a frying pan, sauté together:

| | |
|---|---|
| 1 | Large onion, chopped |
| 2 | Carrots, chopped |
| 2 | Celery stalks, finely chopped |
| 3 | Garlic cloves, minced and rested |
| 1 | Leek, thinly sliced |

Cooked until well done—this adds a lot of flavour to your soups.

Place the vegetables and all juices in a pressure cooker.

Add

| | |
|---|---|
| | Chicken bones (use saved and frozen bones to make a full pot) |
| 2 | Bay leaves |
| ½ t | Whole peppercorns |
| 1 t | Salt |
| 1 t | Thyme |
| 1 T | Parsley |
| 1 L | Chicken broth (Kirkland organic chicken broth is wheat-free) |
| 1 L | Water (as much needed to get up to the fill line) |

Pressure cook for 45 minutes and let the steam release naturally. After 45 minutes, remove and discard the bay leaves and the chicken bones. Add back the chicken meat if desired.

Let cool thoroughly and then place in freezer containers.

This broth can be frozen for up to six months.

Note: This broth becomes the base for many different soups.

# FRENCH ONION SOUP

|         | In a pan, heat over low heat:                                           |
|---------|-------------------------------------------------------------------------|
| 1 T     | Butter                                                                  |
| ¼ c     | Olive oil                                                               |
| Add     |                                                                         |
| 3       | Large onions, sliced                                                    |
|         | Cook the onions until caramelized, about 10 minutes.                    |
|         | Stir into the juices:                                                   |
| 1 T     | Cassava flour                                                           |
| Add     |                                                                         |
| 1 L     | Chicken broth (Kirkland organic chicken broth is wheat-free)            |
| ½ c     | Red wine                                                                |
| ½ t     | Thyme                                                                   |
| ½ t     | Freshly ground black pepper                                             |
|         | Reduce heat to low and cook for 10 minutes.                             |
|         |                                                                         |
|         | Place the soup into onion soup bowls and cover with:                    |
| ¾ c     | Blend of shredded cheeses (cheddar and parmesan)                        |
|         | Bake in the oven at 425° for 10 minutes until the cheese is fully melted.|

# KATELYN'S TURKEY SOUP

|       | In a pan, heat over low heat: |
|-------|-------------------------------|
| ¼ c   | Olive oil                     |

Add and sauté together:

|   |                                  |
|---|----------------------------------|
| 1 | Large onion, chopped             |
| 4 | Garlic cloves, minced and rested |
| 2 | Large carrots, grated            |
| 2 | Celery stalks, chopped           |

Cook until vegetables are nice and soft, and browning.

Place the cooked vegetables in an Instant Pot.

Add

|       |                             |
|-------|-----------------------------|
| 1 jar | *Turkey Bone Broth*         |
| ½ c   | Red lentils                 |
| 1     | Sweet potato, chopped       |
| 1 t   | Thyme                       |
| 1 T   | Parsley                     |
| 1 t   | Sage                        |
| 2     | Bay leaves                  |
| 1 t   | Salt                        |
| ½ t   | Freshly ground black pepper |

Set the Instant Pot to "soup" and add 10 minutes. Let the steam release naturally.

Let cool completely before pouring into freezer containers.

Note: Freeze for up to 6 months.

# MUSHROOM SOUP GB

## Freeze for up to 6 months

|  | In a frying pan, melt: |
| 3 T | Butter |
| Add |  |
| 4 c | Mushrooms, chopped |
|  | Juice of half a lemon |
|  | Cook over medium-high heat until tender. |
| Add |  |
| 1 | Large onion, chopped |
| 2 | Garlic cloves, minced and rested |
|  | Cook until well browned. Stir in until blended: |
| 2–3 T | Cassava flour |
|  | Slowly add, stirring constantly: |
| 1 L | Chicken broth |
| Add |  |
| 3 T | Goat yogurt (Happy Days brand is excellent) |
| 1 t | Salt |
| ¼ t | Freshly ground black pepper |
| 2 T | Sherry or red wine |
| ¼ t | Nutmeg |
| ⅛ t | Thyme |

Take out about a cup of mushrooms.

Using an immersion blender, blend soup until smooth and then add back the mushrooms.

# SPICY CARROT SOUP

|  | In a pan, heat oil: |
| 4 T | Olive oil |
| Add |  |
| 3 | Garlic cloves, minced and rested |
| 5–6 | Large carrots, chopped |
| 1 c | Onion, chopped |
| 1 c | Celery, chopped |
| 1 t | Salt |

Cook the vegetables until soft.

| Add |  |
| 1 T | Orange zest |
| ¼ t | Cumin |
| 1 t | Ginger |
| 3 c | Vegetable broth |
| ¼ t | Freshly ground black pepper |

Bring to a boil and then simmer for 15 to 20 minutes.

Using an immersion blender, blend until smooth.

Let the soup cool completely before pouring into freezer containers.

# TURKEY BONE BROTH GB

---
### Pressure cooker
---

|        | In a pan, heat over low heat:<br>Olive oil |
|--------|-------------------------------------------|
| ¼ c    | Olive oil                                 |

In a frying pan, sauté together:

| 1 | Large onion, chopped |
| 2 | Carrots, chopped |
| 3 | Celery stalks, finely chopped |
| 3 | Garlic cloves, minced and rested |

Place the vegetables in a pressure cooker.

Add
| 1    | Turkey carcass |
| 2    | Bay leaves |
| ½ t  | Whole peppercorns |
| 1 t  | Salt |
| 1 t  | Thyme |
| 1 T  | Parsley |
|      | Water (enough to reach the fill line) |

Pressure cook for 45 minutes, letting the steam release naturally.

Remove and discard the bay leaves and turkey bones. Add back the turkey meat if desired.

Let cool completely before pouring into freezer containers.


Note: This can be used as a base for many of the soups.

# VEGETABLE BROTH

|       | In a large pot, heat oil:                       |
|-------|-------------------------------------------------|
| 3 T   | Olive oil                                       |
| Add   |                                                 |
| 1     | Large onion, chopped                            |
| 3     | Garlic cloves, minced and rested                |

Cook until the onions are browning.

| Add   |                                                 |
|-------|-------------------------------------------------|
| 2 c   | Carrots, chopped                                |
| 2 c   | Parsnips, chopped                               |
| 1     | Large leek, chopped                             |
| 1 c   | Mushrooms, chopped                              |
| 2     | Celery stalks, chopped                          |
| 1     | Large broccoli stem, peeled and chopped         |
| 1 c   | Cabbage, chopped                                |

Cook together until vegetables are soft.

| Add   |                                                   |
|-------|---------------------------------------------------|
| 1 T   | Apple cider vinegar                               |
| 2     | Bay leaves                                        |
| 1 t   | Basil                                             |
| 1 t   | Thyme                                             |
|       | Leftover vegetable water                          |
|       | Water (to make up a total of 3 litres of liquid)  |

Bring to a boil and then turn down to simmer for 1 hour.

Strain out the vegetables.

Let cool completely before putting into freezer containers.

# Sweets and Things

## FOR WHEN YOU WANT SOMETHING SWEET

It's important to have options

It's important to stay with lectin-reduced ingredients so your gut buddies stay happy. They reduce cravings, which helps you stay on track.

Remember, good nutrition is focusing on foods that build and aren't just empty calories.

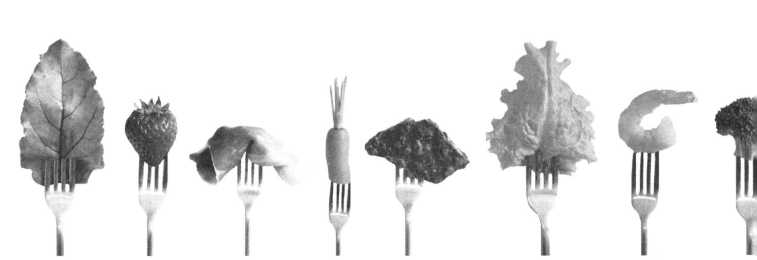

# GINGER SNAP COOKIES

Preheat oven 350° | 10–12 minutes

In a large bowl, stir together dry ingredients:

| | |
|---|---|
| 2 c | Almond flour |
| ¼ t | Salt |
| 1 t | Baking soda |
| 2 t | Ground ginger |
| ¼ t | Nutmeg |
| ¼ t | Cloves |
| ¼ t | Cinnamon |
| ¼ t | Allspice |

In a small bowl, whisk together:

| | |
|---|---|
| ¼ c | Softened butter |
| 1 T | Molasses |
| 1 T | Maple syrup |
| 1 packet | Stevia |
| 1 | Egg |
| 1 t | Vanilla |

Add to the dry ingredients.

Drop batter by the teaspoonful onto an oiled cookie sheet.
Using a fork, flatten cookies slightly.

Bake at 350° for 10 to 12 minutes. Allow to cool before storage.

Note: Include chopped walnuts or other nuts to add variety.

# RAW BROWNIE BITS GB

|       | In a bowl of water, place:                                        |
|-------|-------------------------------------------------------------------|
| 6–8   | Pitted dates                                                      |
|       | Soak for 15 minutes and then chop them in a food processor.       |
| Add   |                                                                   |
| 2 T   | Goat yogurt                                                       |
| 1 t   | Vanilla                                                           |
|       | Bit of salt                                                       |
|       | Process for 30 seconds.                                           |
|       | In a blender, add:                                                |
| 1 c   | Almonds, sliced                                                   |
| ½ c   | Walnuts, chopped                                                  |
| ½ c   | Hemp hearts                                                       |
| 3–4 T | Cacao powder                                                      |

Blend into a fine meal. Add the date mix to the blender.
Blend for 45 to 60 seconds.

Drop batter by the teaspoonful onto an oiled cookie sheet.

Freeze for 20 minutes and then seal in an airtight container.

Note: These are best stored in the freezer—bring them out as you need.

# SINLESS CHOCOLATE CAKE*

## Serves two

|            | In a large bowl, combine: |
|------------|---------------------------|
| 2 T        | Cocoa powder              |
| 1 packet   | Stevia                    |
| 1 T        | Maple syrup               |
| ¼ t        | Baking powder             |

Stir well.

In a small bowl, whisk together:

|            |              |
|------------|--------------|
| 1          | Egg          |
| 1 T        | Coconut milk |
| ½ t        | Vanilla      |

Pour into the cocoa mix and blend well.

Pour into a greased onion soup bowl and microwave for 2 minutes. Turn onto a plate.

Drizzle with:

|            |                                       |
|------------|---------------------------------------|
| 2 T        | Melted almond butter or dark chocolate |

* Inspired by Dr. S. Gundry recipe

# SWEET POTATO WALNUT CAKE

Instant Pot

In a large bowl, combine:

| | |
|---|---|
| 1¼ c | Almond flour |
| ½ c | Cassava flour |
| ¼ c | Coconut flour |
| 1 packet | Stevia |
| ⅛ c | Coconut sugar |
| 2 t | Cinnamon |
| ½ t | Ground ginger |
| ¼ t | Nutmeg |
| ¼ t | Allspice |
| ¼ t | Cloves |
| 1 t | Baking soda |
| ½ t | Salt |

In a small bowl,, combine:

| | |
|---|---|
| 3 | Eggs, whisked |
| ½ c | Sweet potato, mashed |
| ½ c | Goat yogurt |
| 2 T | Avocado oil |
| 2 t | Apple cider vinegar |

Stir well. Mix into the dry ingredients.

Lightly stir into the combined mixture:

| | |
|---|---|
| ⅓ c | Walnuts, chopped |

Pour into a pressure cooker (for creating the steam):

| | |
|---|---|
| ¾ c | Water |

Line a baking dish with parchment paper—be sure the dish fits into the pressure cooker.

Pour batter into the baking dish. Place dish on a rack in the pressure cooker and lay a piece of tin foil on top of it. (It keeps the water from dripping onto the cake).

Set the time for 30 minutes, letting the pressure release naturally and slowly.

Remove the tin foil and baking dish. Carefully remove the parchment paper and cake from the dish. Set on a wire rack to cool.

Note: Keep refrigerated as this cake is very moist.

# Vegetables

## SHOP LOCALLY FOR NUTRIENT-DENSE VEGGIES

Buy at your local farmers' markets

Shopping within 100 miles helps you avoid the added preservatives and tinkering the food industry does to keep food looking fresh. Some of the food industry's practices result in lost potential for nutrient dense food.

Find local farmers to buy from directly when and where you can. Ask a lot of questions about the source of foods. (Unfortunately, some local farmers' markets have been known to resell store-bought foods under the guise of locally grown. Buyer beware!)

Buy vegetables in season and look for as much variety as possible. The winter months make shopping for fresh local root vegetables more difficult. Consider sprouting some on your window ledge for added variety.

**Resistant starches**

A word about resistant starches—they're gut buddies' perfect friends since they're digested more slowly in the gut. Resistant starches don't breakdown entirely; some become short-chain fatty acids on which gut buddies thrive. As well, resistant starches provide both soluble and insoluble fibres. These fibres provide bulk in the intestines and help you feel full longer and provide bulk for proper elimination. Regularly adding resistant starches to meal plans is especially important for folks living with abdominal issues.

Examples of lectin-reduced resistant starches:

Yams, cooked and cold potatoes, taro, parsnips, turnips, jicama, celeriac root, artichokes, sweet potato, plantains and shirataki noodles.

After you feel your gut returning to more normal digestion and elimination, try reintroducing beans and lentils (in pressure-cooker recipes only).

Remember to let your garlic rest for 10 to 15 minutes after it's chopped or minced; this allows the medicinal properties to be their most helpful.

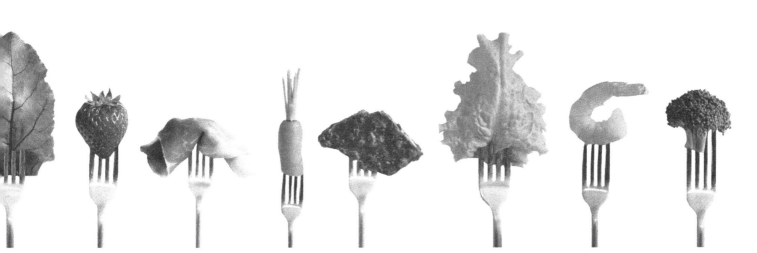

# ASPARAGUS ROASTED

Preheat oven 400° | 10 minutes

|       | Prepare: |
|-------|----------|
|       | Prepare: |
| 2 c   | Asparagus |

Break the stems where they break off naturally and then peel the bottom inch or two to expose the fleshy insides.

In a small bowl, toss asparagus with:

| 2 T | Olive oil |

Sprinkle lightly with:

| ½ t | Salt and freshly ground pepper |

Lay out asparagus on a baking pan. Bake at 400° for 10 minutes or until they pierce easily with a fork. Transfer to a serving dish.

Drizzle with:

| 1 T | Olive oil |

Serve.

Note: Freeze all the unused bottoms; when you've collected 4 cups, make some creamy *Asparagus Soup*.

# BEETS & CARROTS SPICED

Serve with Swiss Steak

| | |
|---|---|
| | In a instant pot: |
| 3/4 c | Water |
| 2 | Medium beets, washed with stems and tails intact |
| | Cook until done, about 10 to 20 minutes depending on the beet size. |
| | Place in a bowl and let cool until they can be handled. Slip off the skins or peel them quickly, and slice. |
| | In a pan, steam: |
| 2 | Medium whole carrots, peeled |
| | Slice them and add to the bowl of beets. |
| | In a small bowl, whisk together: |
| 1 t | Lemon zest |
| 1 | Small shallot, sliced |
| ¼ t | Cumin |
| ¼ t | Maple syrup |
| ¼ c | Pecans or walnuts, chopped |
| 1 t | Parsley |
| | Toss together with the vegetables and serve. |
| | Pairs nicely with *Swiss Steak*. |

Note: Cooking vegetables whole retains more nutrients in the vegetable.

# BLACKBERRY VINEGAR SAUTÉED CABBAGE

## Nice variety

|          | In a frying pan, heat oil:         |
|----------|------------------------------------|
| 2 T      | Olive oil                          |
| Add      |                                    |
| 1        | Red onion, thinly sliced           |
|          | Sauté the onion.                   |
| Add      |                                    |
| 2 c      | Cabbage, thinly sliced             |
| 2 t      | Rosemary                           |
| To taste | Salt                               |
|          | Continue cooking.                  |
| Add      |                                    |
| 2        | Prosciutto ham slices, chopped     |
| 1 T      | Blackberry or raspberry vinegar    |
|          | Stir until heated. Sprinkle with:  |
| ¼ c      | Shredded cheddar cheese            |

Note: This is a wonderful variation for serving cabbage.

# BRUSSELS SPROUTS ROASTED WITH BALSAMIC VINEGAR & LIME

Preheat oven 350° | An unusual twist

In a bowl, toss together:

| | |
|---|---|
| 1 c | Brussels sprouts, cut in half |
| 2 T | Olive oil |

Transfer to a baking pan and bake at 350° until golden. Set aside to cool.

In a small bowl, combine:

| | |
|---|---|
| 1 T | Balsamic vinegar |
| ½ c | Dates, chopped |
| | Juice of a lime |
| | Zest of half a lime |
| 1 t | Garlic, minced and rested |
| ¼ c | Almonds, sliced and toasted |
| To taste | Salt |

Mix well. Add to Brussels sprouts when cooled slightly.

# BRUSSELS SPROUTS WITH LEMON & ALMONDS

A crunchy change

|  | In a frying pan, heat oil: |
|---|---|
| 1 T | Olive oil |
| Add | |
| 1 c | Brussels sprouts, thinly sliced |
|  | Sauté until the Brussels sprouts become slightly browned. |
|  | In a bowl, combine: |
| ½ c | Almonds, thinly chopped |
|  | Juice of a lemon |
| To taste | Salt and freshly ground black pepper |
|  | Pour over Brussels sprouts and toss. Sprinkle with: |
|  | Parmesan cheese, grated |
|  | Serve. |

# CAULIFLOWER FRIED RICE

Excellent potato replacement

|  | In a food processor, place: |
|---|---|
| ⅓ | Cauliflower head |
|  | Process until cauliflower is a rice consistency (or grate for the same results). |
|  | In large frying pan, heat oil on medium-high: |
| 2 T | Olive oil |
| Add | |
| 2 | Small shallots, thinly sliced |
|  | Cook until soft. |
|  | Add the cauliflower rice and cook until lightly browned and translucent. |
| Add | |
| To taste | Salt and freshly ground black pepper |

# CAULIFLOWER RICE CASSEROLE

Great side dish

|  | In a pan, heat oil: |
| --- | --- |
| 2 t | Coconut oil |
| Add |  |
| ½ | Onion, finely chopped |
| 1 t | Turmeric |
| 1 t | Curry |
|  | Cook the onion. |
| Add |  |
| 2 c | Cauliflower rice |
| 1 c | Almonds, slivered |
|  | Cook for 3 to 4 minutes. |
| Add |  |
| 1 c | Cranberries |
| ½ c | Coconut milk |
|  | Continue cooking. |
| Add |  |
| 1 c | Spinach |
|  | Continue cooking until the spinach wilts. |

Note: This is a great side dish.

# CELERIAC/CAULIFLOWER MASHED GB

In a pot cook until soft:

| | |
|---|---|
| 1/2 c | Water |
| ½ | Large cauliflower, sliced |
| 1 | Small celeriac, peeled and sliced |
| 1 | Garlic clove, minced and rested |

Drain

Using an immersion blender, blend to desired consistency.

Add
| | |
|---|---|
| 2 T | Olive oil |

Blend.

Add
| | |
|---|---|
| ¼ c | Chicken broth |
| ½ c | Goat yogurt |

Stir until everything is smooth.

Season with:

| | |
|---|---|
| To taste | Salt and freshly ground black pepper |
| ½ t | Thyme (or other herbs) |

# CELERIAC ROASTED WITH YOGURT DRESSING GB

## Preheat oven 400°

In a bowl, toss together:

| | |
|---|---|
| 2 | Medium celeriac, peeled and sliced into ½-inch thick slices |
| 3 T | Olive oil |
| To taste | Salt and freshly ground black pepper |

Place on a flat pan and bake at 400°, turning over after about 20 minutes. Cook until nice and brown.

**Dressing**

Whisk together:

| | |
|---|---|
| ¼ c | Goat yogurt |
| 1 t | Lime juice |
| ¼ t | Lime zest |
| ¼ t | Thyme |
| ½ T | Parsley |

Drizzle dressing over the celeriac.

Top with:

| | |
|---|---|
| 1 T | Toasted sesame seeds |

Note: This is a great side dish.

# JICAMA FRIES GB

|        | Steam until soft: |
|--------|-------------------|
| ½      | Jicama, cut into ½-inch strips |
|        | Place jicama strips in a baking dish and season with: |
| 2 T    | Olive oil |
| Sprinkle | Chili powder (or any seasonings such as parsley, oregano, basil) |
|        | Blend well. |
|        | Bake at 450° for 10 to 15 minutes. Flip and continue cooking another 10 to 15 minutes. |

Note: Do not burn.

# OVEN-ROASTED BREADED CAULIFLOWER

### Preheat oven 375° | 10–15 minutes

|       | In a bowl, combine: |
|-------|---------------------|
| ½     | Cauliflower, chopped into pieces |
| 1     | Bread bun, crumbled |

Place into a baking dish and toss with:

| 2 T   | Olive oil |
| ¼ t   | Salt and freshly ground black pepper |

Continue tossing and then add:

| 1     | Garlic clove, minced and rested |
| 2 T   | Olive oil |
| 1 t   | Lemon juice |

Bake at 375° for 10 to 15 minutes.

Note: This is a great variation for cauliflower.

# PROSCIUTTO HAM BROCCOLI

## Delicious side dish

|       |                                                                      |
|-------|----------------------------------------------------------------------|
|       | In a skillet, heat oil:                                              |
| 3 T   | Olive oil                                                            |
| Add   |                                                                      |
| 3     | Slices Prosciutto ham, chopped                                      |
|       | Sauté briefly and then remove the meat and set it aside.            |
|       | Steam until light green:                                             |
| ½     | Broccoli, chopped, stem removed                                      |
|       | Add steamed broccoli to skillet along with:                         |
| ¼     | Red pepper, deseeded, peeled and chopped                            |
|       | Cook for a couple minutes.                                           |
| Add   |                                                                      |
|       | Juice of a lemon                                                     |
| 3     | Garlic cloves, minced and rested                                    |
|       | Return ham to the pan and stir well. While still warm, sprinkle with: |
| 2 T   | Grated parmesan cheese                                              |
|       | Serve warm.                                                          |

# ROASTED CARROTS

<hr>

### Preheat oven 375°

<hr>

In a bowl, toss together:

| | |
|---|---|
| 2 T | Olive oil |
| To taste | Salt and freshly ground black pepper |
| 2 c | Carrots, peeled and sliced evenly lengthways |

Sprinkle with:

| | |
|---|---|
| 2 T | Lemon juice |
| ¼ t | Cumin |
| ¼ t | Cinnamon |
| 1 T | Parsley |

Bake at 375° until the carrots are done.

# SWEET POTATO BAKED

<hr>

### Preheat oven 400°

<hr>

In a baking dish, toss together:

| | |
|---|---|
| 2 c | Sweet potato, chopped and cut into ½-inch-thick chunks (no need to peel) |
| 1 T | Olive oil |
| ¼ t | Freshly ground black pepper |
| ½ t | Parsley |

Bake at 400° until done.

# SWEET POTATO FRIES GB

In a bowl, toss together:

| | |
|---|---|
| 1 | Large sweet potato, peeled and sliced into ½-inch-thick fries |
| 1 T | Olive oil |

Add
| | |
|---|---|
| ½ T | Parsley |
| ½ t | Basil |
| ½ t | Oregano |
| To taste | Salt and freshly ground black pepper |

Toss again.

Place on a baking sheet and drizzle with more olive oil.

Bake at 425° for 10 minutes. Turn fries and bake for another 10 minutes or until done.

Note: These are also excellent baked in an air fryer.

Hint: Substitute yam or jicama using the same process for a nice variation.

# SWEET POTATO PANCAKES

Nice for Sunday brunch

In a bowl, combine:

| | |
|---|---|
| 2 c | Sweet potatoes, cooked and mashed |
| 2 | Eggs |
| 1 T | Coconut flour |
| 1 T | Arrowroot flour |
| 1 T | Coconut milk |
| ½ t | Salt |

Mash together and let rest.

In a frying pan, heat oil:

| | |
|---|---|
| 1 T | Olive oil |

Drop mash into pan by the tablespoonful to form small cakes.
Cook until brown. Flip and cook the other side.

Serve with fried eggs and bread buns for a nice Sunday brunch.

# VEGETABLE CHILI

## Instant Pot | Super chili

|  |  |
|---|---|
|  | Prepare beans 24 hours before cooking the chili. |
| **Beans** |  |
|  | In a pot of water, add: |
| 4 c | Black beans |
|  | Soak beans for 24 hours, changing the water a number of times. |
|  | Place in a pot and cover with boiling water and cook until soft, adding water as needed. |
| **Chili** |  |
|  | In an Instant Pot, combine: |
| 2 T | Olive oil |
| 1 | Medium onion, chopped |
| 4 | Garlic cloves, minced and rested |
|  | Turn Instant Pot to "sauté" and cook. |
| Add |  |
| 2 | Medium carrots, chopped |
| 2 | Small parsnips, chopped |
| 2 c | Mushrooms, chopped |
|  | Sauté vegetables until browned. |
| Add |  |
| 4 c | Black beans, pre-cooked (as above) |
| 6 | Roma tomatoes, fresh or frozen |
| ½ c | *Katelyn's Tomato Sauce* |
| 1½ c | Water |
| 2 T | Molasses |
| 2 t | Cumin |
| ½ t | Salt |
| ½ t | Freshly ground black pepper |
| ⅛ t | Cayenne pepper |
| ⅛ t | Chili powder |
|  | Turn the Instant Pot to "beans" and add 15 minutes. Set the lid tightly and cook, letting steam release naturally. |

Note: Freeze in portion sizes for quick meals.

# VEGETABLE CRISPS

### Preheat oven 400° | 20 minutes

In a bowl, combine:

| | |
|---|---|
| 3 c | Broccoli, finely chopped |
| 1 c | Carrots, shredded |
| 3 T | Parmesan cheese, grated |
| 2 T | Cassava flour |
| 2 | Eggs |
| To taste | Salt and freshly ground black pepper |

Mix well.

Add batter by tablespoonful onto a baking pan.

Bake at 400° for 20 minutes. Flip and cook an additional 10 minutes until crisps are golden brown.

Note: These are great as a snack or served with soup as a bread replacement.

# VEGETABLE LASAGNA

Preheat oven 350° | 1 hour

|  | In a skillet, heat oil: |
| 1 T | Olive oil |
| Add | |
| 1 | Large onion, chopped |
|  | Cook the onion. |
| Add | |
| 1 lb | Ground bison or beef |
|  | Brown the meat to crumbling. |
| Add | |
| 1 t | Oregano |
| 1 t | Basil |
|  | Set aside. Slice very thinly lengthways: |
| 2 | Large sweet potatoes |
|  | Set aside. |

**Build lasagna**

In a baking dish, begin layering. Cover bottom with:

*Katelyn's Tomato Sauce*

Add other ingredients:

| ¼ c | Crumbled, cooked meat (as above) |
|  | Sweet potato slices (laid out and not overlapping) |
| ½ c | Spinach, a little at a time |
| 2 T | Grated parmesan cheese |

Start over with next layer, beginning with a layer of tomato sauce.
Continue until baking dish is filled and all ingredients used.

Top with:

| ½ c | Shredded mozzarella cheese |
| 2 T | Grated parmesan cheese |

Bake at 350° for 1 hour. Increase to 400° and brown the cheese on top.

# REFERENCES

In this journey, I've discovered some excellent high-quality products
I would like to share with you

Cosman & Webb Townships Organic in Bury, Quebec coswebb.ca

They sell an excellent quality maple syrup they will ship to your door. They use no toxic chemicals in cleaning the equipment and syrup lines. I felt no ill effects from using their product. Venturi Schulze referred them to me.

Dr. Steven Gundry, author of the five Plant Paradox books gundrymd.com

Fieldstone Organics in Armstrong, BC fieldstoneorganics.ca

A co-operative started in 2000, with growers and farmers in the Okanagan. Great bulk purchasing.

Grass Root Dairies in Salmon Arm, BC grassrootdairies.com

All A2 cheeses. Canada first 100% grass-fed registered dairy farm. They feed no grains to their cows.

Hardy Hills Farm in Chase, BC hardyhillsfarm.com

A sustainable, regenerative pasture-based farm with grass-fed and grass-finished beef, lamb, pork and chicken. They also have a very productive vegetable garden and pasture-raised eggs.

Rancho Vignola in Vernon, BC ranchovignola.com

An excellent wholesale company that sells organic nuts and seeds. I've used them for years and have always been impressed with their service and quality. It does require one-time annual purchases.

Venturi Schulze Vineyard in Cobble Hill, BC on Vancouver Island venturischulze.com

We discovered them while doing a wine tour on Vancouver Island. They have a wine and balsamic vinegar tasting room. Their balsamic vinegar is the secret ingredient in my tomato sauce and baked beans. They now have a maple balsamic vinegar that will leave you breathless.

On the following page you'll find a shopping list I created based on Dr. S. Gundry's Yes List. My thinking is to focus on the foods we can enjoy. This list will help you make sure your pantry remains well stocked with the required ingredients for these recipes.

Photography: Nell Miller

# GROCERY LIST

## FOODS THAT DO NOT CAUSE INFLAMMATION

**OILS**
Avocado
Coconut
Ghee
Olive
MCT
Sesame

**BAKING**
72% chocolate
Apple cider vinegar
Avocado mayonnaise
Olives
Miso
Soup stock

**FLOUR**
Almond
Arrowroot
Cassava
Coconut
Sorghum
Tapioca
Tigernut flour

**GRAINS & PASTA**
Miracle Noodle
Fettuccini
Rice
Spinach spaghetti
Millet

**SEEDS & NUTS**
Almonds
Flax seed
Hemp seeds
Pecans
Pistachios
Poppyseed
Psyllium husks
Sesame seeds
Walnuts

**CANNED FISH WILD**
Salmon
Sardines

**MEAT & PROTEIN**
Bison
Chicken
Prosciutto ham
Turkey
Omega-3/pastured eggs

**FISH**
Salmon
Cod
Shrimp
Snapper

**DAIRY & ALTERNATES**
Buffalo mozzarella
Butter
Coconut milk/yogurt
Goat cheese/yogurt
Organic heavy cream
Parmigiano reggiano
Vintage cheese

**VEGETABLES**
Arugula
Asparagus
Beets
Broccoli
Brussels sprouts
Cabbage
Carrots
Cauliflower
Celeriac
Celery
Cilantro
Garlic
Jicama
Kale
Kohlrabi
Leeks
Lettuce leaf
Mushrooms
Onions and greens
Parsnips
Portobello
Radicchio
Romaine
Rutabaga
Spinach
Sweet potato
Swiss chard
Yam

**SPICES**
Allspice
Basil
Bay leaf
Cayenne
Celery seed
Chili powder
Cinnamon
Cloves
Curry
Ginger
Mustard
Nutmeg
Oregano
Paprika
Parsley
Peppercorn
Rosemary
Sage
Thyme
Turmeric

**MISCELLANEOUS**
Almond butter
Baking soda
Balsamic vinegar
Coconut aminos
Capers
Fish sauce
Molasses
Nutter baking powder
Pickling spice
Poultry seasoning
Salt
Sriracha sauce
Worcestershire
Yeast

**FRUIT**
Avocado
Dates
Limes
Lemons
Fruit in season

**Note**
A1 milk is generally from Holstein cows and A2 milk is from the European brown cow. If you experience digestive discomfort with milk products, stick to A2 milk products and limit dairy to cheeses and butter, as casein is reduced in the fat. Or switch your shopping patterns to goat cheese, sheep cheese or water buffalo cheese (which is not always easy to find).

# INDEX

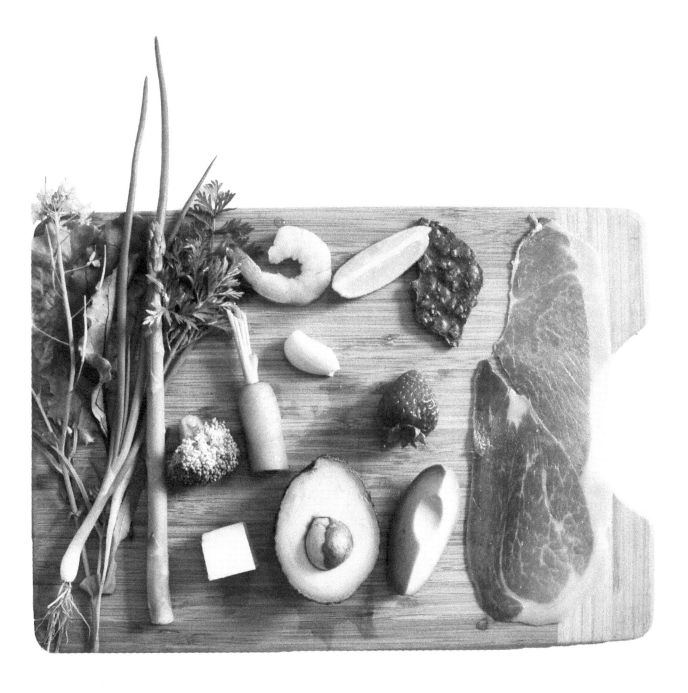

# ABOUT THE AUTHORS

## Katelyn (Deb) Miller RN, Dipl.P.H., BSN

I pursued a career path in allopathic medicine in nursing for sixteen years before I made abrupt changes in my life. Having ill health and not finding the answers for better health were part of my decision to leave nursing.

My best decision was becoming an organic master gardener. The program took three winters of study and propelled Reg and I in a new direction of thought and awareness.

Indeed, there have been many "aha" moments. The connection I made between what makes good soil that creates nutrient-dense food and what creates a great microbiome in the body was the reason for this journey into nutrition.

Creating a cookbook seemed like a very logical next step.

Reg and I live in rural BC; we see our retirement as the beginning of the next chapter.

To quote Steve Solomon in *The Intelligent Gardner*, "I have invented a word to describe my lifestyle: *vegetableatarianism*. The word does not mean that animal foods are excluded. A vegetableatarian is someone who's trying to repair the damage caused by harmful food addictions by eating mostly vegetables, cooked and raw."

## Linda Thompson

I started my new healthy journey one year ago. The improvements have been fantastic and I feel less stiffness and arthritic pain. The best part is experiencing no brain fog and feeling that I'm communicating better.

The time my sister, Deb, and I spent creating new recipes was interesting and very encouraging as we began to experience a new way of health. We spent many months creating new ideas for our menu plans. The best part was gardening and learning to grow different vegetables and herbs, and also grapes. It was very satisfying to create flower garden areas that attract beneficial pollinators.

Deb taught me how to create a good compost and improve my soil to maximize its vitamin and mineral content. Having the energy to creatively design my yard and pursue my artistic skills, quilting and painting has been wonderful.

I enjoy this new level of energy each day because of the changes I made in my food decisions. Daily, I spend time reading gardening books, gathering information and viewing Dr. S. Gundry's YouTube videos so I can keep improving my health.

I am seventy now, with the energy to enjoy my favourite pastimes. I look forward to every day.

# FEEDBACK

### Reg Miller

Congratulations to Katelyn and Linda for creating this first of what I believe will be ongoing revision of recipes and health ideas.

This book came out of a somewhat random process of information gleaned through the new reality of the internet—the level of available information is quite stunning— and more recently from *The Plant Paradox* by Dr. Gundry, a very compelling podcast with Dr. S. Gundry and Dr. J. Mercola, and the work of Dr. Zack Bush.

Our understanding comes out of a couple of long-held vital assumptions: "we are what we eat," and "food is medicine and medicine is food." We discovered the amazing information about the gut microbiome and the importance of eating not just for our bodies but also our billions of gut bacteria. That is the story. This set of recipes is an attempt to help you eat for health.

Although this book is not a weight-loss manifesto, my story is compelling evidence of its efficacy. Now in my 65th year, I start my retirement with having lost 90 pounds and kept it off.

I have been the coaxed participant in this story for just over a year now. I must say that I have personally eaten every recipe in this book—and, may I add, the kitchen helper in much of it. Without hesitation, I give it the Reggie-Approved Award of Excellence.

For someone like me, who can find recipes to be overwhelming,
I appreciate the step-by-step instructions —Nell Miller

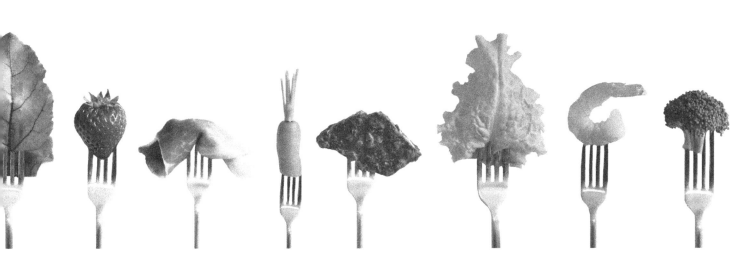

CPSIA information can be obtained
at www.ICGtesting.com
Printed in the USA
LVHW060504270422
717356LV00010B/228